PRACTICE GUIDELINE

FOR THE

TREATMENT OF

PATIENTS WITH

PANIC DISORDER

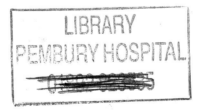
American Psychiatric Association

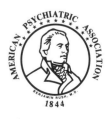

Copyright © 1998 American Psychiatric Association
ALL RIGHTS RESERVED
Manufactured in the United States of America on acid-free paper
First Edition
01 00 99 98   4 3 2 1

American Psychiatric Association
1400 K Street, N.W., Washington, DC   20005
ISSN 1067-8743
ISBN 0-89042-311-3

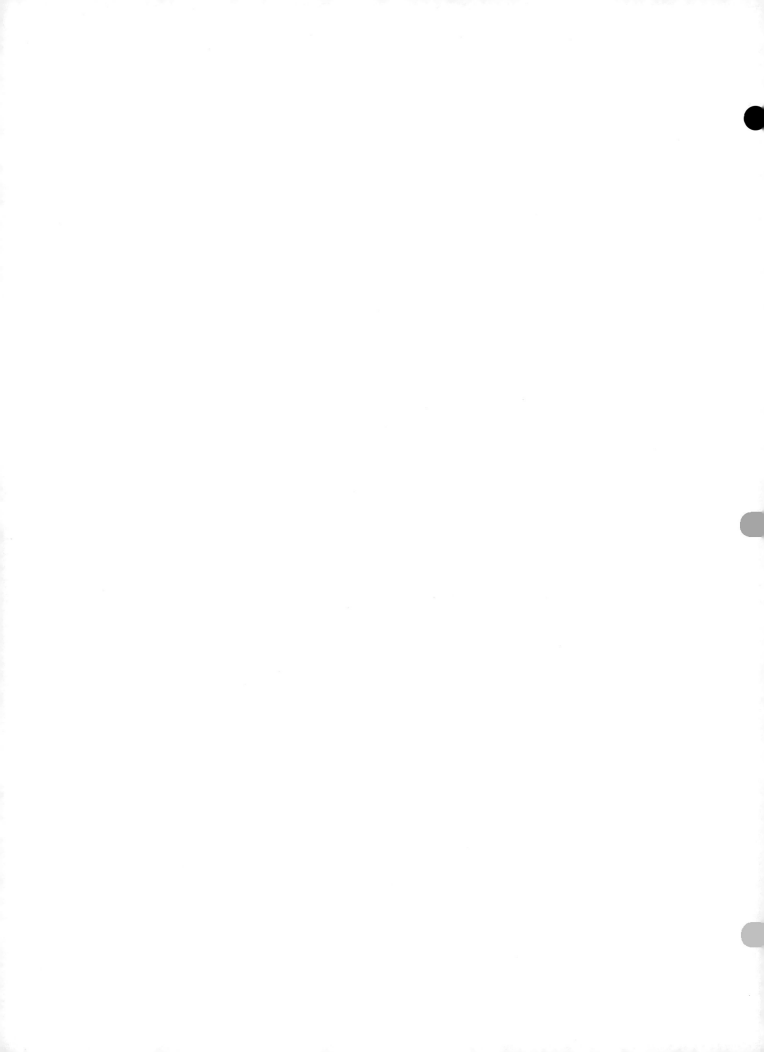

TABLE OF CONTENTS

STATEMENT OF INTENT

This guideline is not intended to be construed or to serve as a standard of medical care. Standards of medical care are determined on the basis of all clinical data available for an individual case and are subject to change as scientific knowledge and technology advance and patterns evolve. These parameters of practice should be considered guidelines only. Adherence to them will not ensure a successful outcome in every case, nor should they be construed as including all proper methods of care aimed at the same results. The ultimate judgment regarding a particular clinical procedure or treatment plan must be made by the psychiatrist in light of the clinical data presented by the patient and the diagnostic and treatment options available.

This practice guideline has been developed by psychiatrists who are in active clinical practice. In addition, some contributors are primarily involved in research or other academic endeavors. It is possible that through such activities some contributors have received income related to treatments discussed in this guideline. A number of mechanisms are in place to minimize the potential for producing biased recommendations due to conflicts of interest. The guideline has been extensively reviewed by members of APA as well as by representatives from related fields. Contributors and reviewers have all been asked to base their recommendations on an objective evaluation of the available evidence. Any contributor or reviewer who has a potential conflict of interest that may bias (or appear to bias) his or her work has been asked to notify the APA Office of Research. This potential bias is then discussed with the work group chair and the chair of the Steering Committee on Practice Guidelines. Further action depends on the assessment of the potential bias.

This practice guideline was approved in December 1997 and was published in May 1998.

INTRODUCTION

This guideline summarizes data to inform the psychiatrist of the care of patients with panic disorder. It begins at the point where the psychiatrist has diagnosed an adult patient as suffering from this disorder according to the criteria in DSM-IV (1) and has evaluated the patient for the existence of coexisting mental disorders. It also assumes that the psychiatrist or other physician has evaluated the patient for general medical conditions or other factors that may be causing or exacerbating the panic or that may affect its treatment. The guideline also briefly addresses issues specific to the treatment of panic disorder in children and adolescents.

The purpose of this guideline is to assist the psychiatrist in caring for a patient with panic disorder. It should be noted that many patients have conditions that cannot be completely described by the DSM-IV diagnostic category. The psychiatrist caring for a patient with panic disorder should consider, but not be limited to, the treatments recommended in this practice guideline. Psychiatrists care for patients with panic disorders in many different settings and serve a variety of functions; the recommendations in this guideline are primarily intended for psychiatrists who provide, or coordinate, the overall care of the patient with panic disorder.

DEVELOPMENT PROCESS

This practice guideline was developed under the auspices of the Steering Committee on Practice Guidelines. The process is detailed in a document available from the APA Office of Research, the "APA Guideline Development Process." Key features of the process include the following:

- a comprehensive literature review (description follows) and development of evidence tables
- initial drafting by a work group that included psychiatrists with clinical and research expertise in panic disorder
- the production of multiple drafts with widespread review, in which 20 organizations and over 100 individuals submitted comments (see section VII)
- approval by the APA Assembly and Board of Trustees
- planned revisions at 3- to 5-year intervals

The following computerized searches of relevant literature were conducted.

The first literature search was conducted by using MEDLINE and Psychological Abstracts, for the period of 1980–1994. The key words for the search were "panic disorder," "agoraphobia," "drug treatment," "non-drug treatment," and "combined modality treatment." A total of 825 citations were found.

A second search was conducted in MEDLINE for the period of 1980–1994 and used the key words "panic disorder" and "tricyclics," "MAO inhibitors," "benzodiazepines," "SSRI's and anticonvulsants," "behavioral and/or cognitive," "all other psychotherapy/psychoanalysis," and "children without adults and combined child and adult." In Psychological Abstracts the key words "panic disorder" and "psychosocial treatment" were used.

A third search was completed in MEDLINE for the period 1992–1996 and used the following key words: "panic disorder," "agoraphobia," "antidepressive agents," "tricyclic," "MAO inhibitors," "benzodiazepine," "anti-anxiety agents," "anticonvulsants," "behavior therapy," "psychotherapy/psychoanalysis," "children," and "psychosocial treatment."

I. Summary of Recommendations

A. CODING SYSTEM

Each recommendation is identified as falling into one of three categories of endorsement, indicated by a bracketed Roman numeral following the statement. The three categories represent varying levels of clinical confidence regarding the recommendation:

[I] recommended with substantial clinical confidence.
[II] recommended with moderate clinical confidence.
[III] may be recommended on the basis of individual circumstances.

B. GENERAL CONSIDERATIONS

Panic disorder, with or without agoraphobia, is a common psychiatric illness that can have a chronic course and be associated with significant morbidity. The care of patients with panic disorder involves a comprehensive array of approaches that are designed to reduce the frequency and severity of panic episodes, reduce morbidity, and improve patient functioning [I]. Modalities for which there is considerable evidence of efficacy in the treatment of panic disorder include psychotherapy, specifically cognitive behavioral therapies, and pharmacotherapy [I]. Other psychotherapies, including psychodynamic, are widely employed in conjunction with medication and/or elements of cognitive behavioral therapies on the basis of a clinical consensus that they are effective for some patients [II]. Considerations for choosing specific treatments among the various options are presented.

1. Choice of treatment setting

For most patients with panic disorder, treatment can be conducted on an outpatient basis and rarely requires hospitalization [I]. Examples of patients who may require inpatient treatment include individuals with comorbid depression who are at risk of suicide attempts or patients with comorbid substance use disorders who require detoxification.

Sometimes the first contact between patient and psychiatrist occurs in the emergency room or hospital to which a patient has been admitted for an acute panic episode. The psychiatrist may be able to make the diagnosis of panic disorder and initiate treatment in this setting after general medical conditions have been ruled out.

2. Formulation of a treatment plan

A comprehensive general medical and psychiatric evaluation should precede treatment to determine whether potential general medical and substance-induced conditions may be causing the panic symptoms, complicate treatment, or require specific interventions, especially with a patient who has a new onset of symptoms [I]. In addition, the assessment of developmental factors, psychosocial stressors and conflicts, social supports, and general living situation will aid the treatment [I]. The psychiatrist's evaluation of the patient's condition and the intended treatment should guide the choice of laboratory and diagnostic studies [I].

3. Psychiatric management

Psychiatric management forms the foundation of psychiatric treatment for patients with panic disorder and should be instituted for all patients in combination with specific treatments, such as medications and psychotherapy. The following are important components of psychiatric management for patients with panic disorder [I]: establishing and maintaining a therapeutic alliance; educating and reassuring the patient concerning panic disorder; evaluating particular symptoms and monitoring them over time; evaluating types and severity of functional impairment; identifying and addressing comorbid conditions; working with other health professionals; educating family members and enlisting their help when appropriate; enhancing treatment compliance; and working with the patient to address early signs of relapse. Many patients with panic disorder require a reliable treatment relationship because they relapse or have partial responses and benefit from extended periods of treatment, or because they intensely fear abandonment. For these reasons, it is helpful to be able to assure the patient of the continued availability of his or her psychiatrist.

4. Choice of treatment modalities to be used in conjunction with psychiatric management

Psychotherapy, specifically panic-focused cognitive behavioral therapy (CBT), and medications have both been shown to be effective treatments for panic disorder [I]. There is no convincing evidence that one modality is superior for all patients or for particular subpopulations of patients. The choice between psychotherapy and pharmacotherapy depends on an individualized assessment of the efficacy, benefits, and risks of each modality and the patient's personal preferences (including costs) [I]. In every case, the patient should be fully informed by the psychiatrist about the availability and relative advantages and disadvantages of CBT, antipanic medications, and other forms of treatment.

a. Cognitive behavioral therapy and other psychotherapies

CBT encompasses a range of treatments, each consisting of several elements, including psychoeducation, continuous panic monitoring, development of anxiety management skills, cognitive restructuring, and in vivo exposure. In practice, the types of therapy encompassed by CBT are often quite diverse. It is unknown whether certain elements are more effective for all patients or for specific patients. The efficacy of CBT for the treatment of panic disorder is supported by extensive and high-quality data. Other psychotherapies may be considered in conjunction with psychiatric management [III], but supplementation with (or replacement by) either CBT or an antipanic medication should be strongly considered if there is no significant improvement within 6–8 weeks.

b. Pharmacotherapy

There are four classes of medications that have been shown to be effective: selective serotonin reuptake inhibitors (SSRIs), tricyclic antidepressants (TCAs), benzodiazepines, and monoamine oxidase inhibitors (MAOIs) [I]. Medications from all four classes have been found to have roughly comparable efficacy [II]. Choosing a medication from among these classes is generally guided by considerations of adverse effects and the physician's understanding of the patient's personal preferences (including costs) and other aspects of the clinical situation [I]. For many patients, SSRIs are likely to have the most favorable balance of efficacy and adverse effects. Although SSRIs carry a risk of sexual side effects, they lack the cardiovascular side effects, anticholinergic side effects, and toxicity associated with overdose that occur with TCAs and MAOIs. SSRIs also lack the potential for physiologic dependency associated with benzodiazepines. TCAs can be tolerated by most patients, although generally not as well as SSRIs. The risks of cardiovascular and anticholinergic side effects of TCAs should be considered, especially for the elderly or patients with general medical problems. Benzodiazepines may be used preferentially in situations in which very rapid control of symptoms is critical (e.g., the patient is about to quit school, lose a job, or require hospitalization). However, the risks of long-term benzodiazepine use, including physiologic dependence, should also be considered. Benzodiazepine use is generally contraindicated for patients with a history of substance use disorder. Although MAOIs are effective, they are generally reserved for patients who do not respond to other treatments because of the risk of hypertensive crises and necessary dietary restrictions. SSRIs are likely to be more expensive than TCAs or benzodiazepines because of the lack of generic preparations.

5. Other treatment considerations

a. Combined medication and psychotherapy

Studies comparing the efficacy of combined antipanic medication and CBT with the efficacy of either modality alone have produced conflicting results. Currently, it is not possible to identify which patients might benefit more from combination therapy. Combined antipanic medication and CBT may be especially useful for patients with severe agoraphobia and those who show an incomplete response [III].

b. Determining the length of treatment

With either CBT or antipanic medication, the acute phase of treatment lasts approximately 12 weeks [II]. After this time, many clinicians reduce the frequency of CBT and then gradually discontinue treatment when the patient is judged to be stable. It is not known whether a second round of CBT is effective for patients who relapse or whether "booster" CBT sessions may prevent relapse.

If a medication has been used, a trial of discontinuation may be attempted after 12–18 months of maintenance therapy if the patient has experienced significant or full improvement [III]. Many patients will partially or fully relapse when medication is discontinued and may benefit from prolonged periods of treatment [III]. Although data on the percentage of patients that remain well after medication discontinuation have been widely divergent, evidence suggests that it is between 30% and 45% (2). Patients who relapse are generally given medication again and/or offered CBT. Patients who remain panic free should be encouraged to contact their psychiatrists in the future at the first sign of the reemergence of panic attacks.

Patients who show no improvement within 6–8 weeks with a particular treatment should be reevaluated with regard to diagnosis, the need for a different treatment, or the need for a combined treatment approach [III]. Patients who do not respond as expected to medication or CBT or who have repeated relapses should be evaluated for possible addition of a psychodynamic or other psychotherapeutic intervention.

c. Use of benzodiazepines for early symptom control, in combination with another treatment modality

It may take several weeks of treatment before patients begin to experience noticeable benefits from either CBT or pharmacotherapy. For some patients with severe panic attacks or high levels of anticipatory anxiety, concomitant benzodiazepine use may be helpful [III]. It may be appropriate to minimize the dose and duration when benzodiazepines are used in this manner, because of potential risks (e.g., physiologic dependence).

d. Comorbidities and other clinical features influencing treatment

Comorbid psychiatric illness, concurrent general medical illnesses, and certain demographic or psychosocial features of patients with panic disorder may have important influences on treatment. Prevalent comorbid psychiatric factors that should be considered include suicidality, substance use, mood disorders, other anxiety disorders, personality disorders, and significant dysfunction in personal, social, or vocational areas. Specific psychosocial therapies (including psychodynamic psychotherapy) may be useful to address comorbid disorders or environmental or psychosocial stressors in patients with panic disorder and are frequently used in conjunction with CBT and/or antipanic medications. Important general medical conditions that may be seen with, or confused with, panic disorder include an array of cardiovascular, pulmonary, neurologic, endocrinologic, and gastrointestinal conditions. Special treatment considerations are necessary for pediatric and geriatric patients with panic disorder. Details concerning the influence of these factors on the treatment of patients with panic disorder are found in section V.

II. DISEASE DEFINITION, NATURAL HISTORY, AND EPIDEMIOLOGY

A. DIAGNOSIS OF PANIC DISORDER

The essential features of panic disorder consist of a mixture of characteristic signs and symptoms that persist for at least 1 month. The symptoms include recurrent panic attacks and persistent concern about having another attack or worry about the implications and consequences of the attacks. Panic attacks are discrete periods of intense fear or discomfort, accompanied by at least four of the 13 somatic or cognitive symptoms defined by DSM-IV. An attack has an abrupt onset and reaches a peak usually within 10 minutes. It is often accompanied by a sense of imminent danger and an urge to escape.

Panic disorder must be distinguished from other conditions that can have panic symptoms as an associated feature. These conditions include other mental disorders (e.g., specific phobias, post-traumatic stress disorder, or separation anxiety disorder), the direct effects of substances, including over-the-counter medications (e.g., caffeine or stimulants), withdrawal from a substance (e.g., withdrawal from sedative-hypnotics), or certain general medical conditions (e.g., hyperthyroidism). For further discussion of these issues, see DSM-IV.

B. SPECIFIC FEATURES OF PANIC DISORDER

1. Cross-sectional issues

There are a number of important clinical and psychosocial features to consider in a cross-sectional evaluation. First, because there is such variance in the types and duration of attacks that may occur with panic disorder, the psychiatrist should consider other possible diagnoses. The psychiatrist should assess the patient for the presence of life-threatening behaviors, the degree to which the panic disorder interferes with the patient's ability to conduct his or her daily routine or to care for self and others, and the presence of a substance use disorder or a depressive disorder.

2. Longitudinal issues

Because of the variable nature of panic disorder, it is necessary to consider a number of longitudinal issues when evaluating the patient. These include the fluctuations in this chronic condition, the development of complications, and the response to prior treatments.

C. NATURAL HISTORY AND COURSE

Several types of panic attacks may occur. The most common is the unexpected attack, defined as one not associated with a known situational trigger. Individuals may also experience situationally predisposed panic attacks (which are more likely to occur in certain situations but do not necessarily occur there) or situationally bound attacks (which occur almost immediately on exposure to a situational trigger). Other types of panic attacks include those that occur in particular emotional contexts, those involving limited symptoms, and nocturnal attacks.

Patients with panic disorder may also have agoraphobia, in which case they experience anxiety and avoidance of places or situations where escape or help may be unavailable if they have panic symptoms. Typical situations eliciting agoraphobia include traveling on buses, subways, or other public transportation and being on bridges, in tunnels, or far from home. Many patients who develop agoraphobia find that situational attacks become more common than unexpected attacks.

Panic attacks vary in their frequency and intensity. It is not uncommon for an individual to experience numerous moderate attacks for months at a time or to experience frequent attacks daily for a short period (e.g., a week), with months separating subsequent periods of attack.

Individuals with panic disorder commonly have anxiety about the recurrence of panic attacks or symptoms or about the implications or consequences. Panic disorder, especially with agoraphobia, may lead to the loss or disruption of interpersonal relationships, especially as individuals struggle with the impairment or loss of social role functioning and the issue of responsibility for symptoms.

Examples of the disrupting nature of panic disorder include the fear that an attack is the indicator of a life-threatening illness despite medical evaluation indicating otherwise or the fear that an attack is a sign of emotional weakness. Some individuals experience the attacks as so severe that they take such actions as quitting a job to avoid a possible attack. Others may become so anxious that they eventually avoid most activities outside their homes. Evidence from one naturalistic follow-up study of patients in a tertiary-care setting suggests that at 4–6 years posttreatment about 30% of individuals are well, 40%–50% are improved but symptomatic, and the remaining 20%–30% have symptoms that are the same or slightly worse (3, 4).

D. EPIDEMIOLOGY AND ASSOCIATED FEATURES

Epidemiologic data collected from a variety of countries have documented similarities in lifetime prevalence (1.6%–2.2%), age at first onset (20s), higher risk in females (about twofold), and symptom patterns of panic disorder (5). While the full-blown syndrome is usually not present until early adulthood, limited symptoms often occur much earlier. Several investigators have documented cases of panic disorder prepubertally (6).

One-third to one-half of individuals diagnosed with panic disorder in community samples also have agoraphobia, although a much higher rate of agoraphobia is encountered in clinical samples (5). Among individuals with panic disorder, the lifetime prevalence of major depression is 50%–60% (7). For individuals with both panic disorder and depression, the onset of depression precedes the onset of panic disorder in one-third of this population, while the onset of depression coincides with or follows the onset of panic disorder in the remaining two-thirds. Approximately one-third of patients with panic disorder are depressed when they present for treatment (7).

Epidemiologic studies have clearly documented the morbidity associated with panic disorder. In the Epidemiologic Catchment Area study, subjects with panic symptoms or disorders, as compared to other disorders, were the most frequent users of emergency medical services and were more likely to be hospitalized for physical problems (8). Patients with panic disorder, especially with comorbid depression, were at higher risk for suicide attempts (9), impaired social and marital functioning, use of psychoactive medication, and substance abuse (10).

Family studies using direct interviews of relatives and family history studies have shown that panic disorder is highly familial. Results from studies conducted in different countries (United States, Belgium, Germany, Australia) have shown that the median risk of panic disorder is eight times as high in the first-degree relatives of probands with panic disorder as in the relatives of control subjects (11). A recent family data analysis showed that forms with early onsets (at age 20 or before) were the most familial, carrying a more than 17 times greater risk (12). Results from twin studies have suggested a genetic contribution to the disorder (13, 14).

III. TREATMENT PRINCIPLES AND ALTERNATIVES

A. PSYCHIATRIC MANAGEMENT

Psychiatric management consists of a comprehensive array of activities and interventions that should be instituted by psychiatrists for all patients with panic disorder, in combination with specific treatment modalities. Patients with panic disorder frequently fear that panic attacks represent catastrophic medical events. In addition, they may live in a nearly constant state of apprehension and may be severely limited by phobic avoidance. For such reasons, reassurance, education, and support are important components of psychiatric management, along with accurate diagnosis that takes into account all the elements of a patient's individual symptom pattern. The psychiatrist should help the patient cope with the effects that panic disorder sometimes has on family members and with the possibility that the disorder may be chronic, requiring long-term treatment.

The specific components of psychiatric management include performing a diagnostic evaluation; evaluating the particular symptoms; evaluating types and severity of functional impairment of the individual patient; establishing and maintaining a therapeutic alliance; monitoring the patient's psychiatric status; providing education to the patient and, when appropriate, to the family about panic disorder; working with nonpsychiatric physicians the patient consults; enhancing treatment compliance; and working with the patient to address early signs of relapse.

1. Performing a diagnostic evaluation

Patients with panic symptoms should receive a thorough diagnostic evaluation both to determine whether a diagnosis of panic disorder is warranted and to reveal the presence of other psychiatric or general medical conditions. Evaluation of a patient with panic disorder frequently involves a number of physicians. The psychiatrist with responsibility for the care of the patient should oversee the evaluation. The general principles and components of a complete psychiatric evaluation have been outlined in the American Psychiatric Association's *Practice Guideline for Psychiatric Evaluation of Adults* (15). This should include a history of the present illness and current symptoms; past psychiatric history; general medical history and history of substance use disorders; personal history (e.g., psychological development, response to life transitions and major life events); social, occupational, and family history; review of the patient's medications; review of systems; mental status examination; physical examination; and diagnostic tests as indicated.

2. Evaluating particular symptoms

Although patients with panic disorder share common features of the illness, there are important interindividual differences. The frequency of panic attacks varies widely among patients, and the constellation of symptoms for each attack also differs. Some patients complain, for example, of attacks that primarily involve cardiovascular symptoms, such as palpitations, chest pain, and paresthesia, while others are more overwhelmed by cognitive symptoms, such as depersonalization and the fear of "losing one's mind." The amount of anticipatory anxiety and the degree of phobic avoidance also vary from patient to patient. Many patients with panic disorder are not highly avoidant; at the opposite extreme are patients who will not leave the house without a trusted companion. It is critical to be sensitive to these individual differences in the elements of panic disorder among patients for two reasons. First, it is important for the patient to feel that the psychiatrist understands accurately the patient's individual experience of panic. Second, treatment may be influenced by the particular constellation of symptoms and other problems of a given patient.

Therefore, it is important to carefully assess the frequency and nature of a patient's panic attacks. It is helpful for patients to monitor their panic attacks, using techniques such as keeping a daily diary, in order to gather data regarding the relationship of panic symptoms to internal stimuli (e.g., emotions) and external stimuli (e.g., substances, particular situations or settings). Such monitoring can be therapeutic.

3. Evaluating types and severity of functional impairment

The degree of functional impairment varies considerably among patients with panic disorder. It is increasingly recognized that resolution of panic attacks, even though they are the core symptom of panic disorder, may be insufficient to warrant the term "clinical remission." As already mentioned, some patients have such high levels of anticipatory anxiety that even when the panic attacks are gone they continue to live restricted lives because of fear. Varying levels of phobic avoidance also determine the degree of impairment experienced by patients with panic disorder. The avoidance of common situations and places, such as driving, restaurants, shopping malls, and elevators, is a cardinal symptom of panic disorder and obviously leads to considerable inability to function in both social and work roles. Sometimes a patient is more focused on the attacks themselves and relegates phobic avoidance to secondary importance. There are situations in which phobic avoidance becomes such a routine part of the patient's life that both the patient and the family are actually reluctant to see it remit. A patient who is homebound because of panic disorder, for example, may have assumed all of the household chores for the family for years. Remission of this kind of phobic avoidance leads to the desire to engage in activities outside of the home, thus leaving a gap. Without recognizing this, family members can tacitly undermine a potentially successful treatment to avoid disrupting their ingrained patterns. In dealing with phobic avoidance and the range of functional impairment seen in patients with panic disorder it is critical to determine exactly what the patient defines as a satisfactory outcome. The patient should be encouraged to define a desirable level of functioning for himself or herself. Treatment of panic disorder should include substantial effort to alleviate or minimize phobic avoidance. Even after the panic attacks have subsided, the patient may continue to have significant limitations in activities that need to be addressed in treatment.

4. Establishing and maintaining a therapeutic alliance

By the very nature of the illness, many patients with panic disorder are extremely anxious about all treatment interventions. Panic disorder is usually a chronic, long-term condition for which adherence to a treatment plan is important. Hence, a strong treatment alliance is crucial. It is often the case that the treatment of panic disorder involves asking the patient to do things that may be frightening and uncomfortable, such as confronting phobic situations. Here again, a strong treatment alliance is necessary to support the patient in doing these things. Patients with panic disorder are generally very sensitive to separations and need to know that the psychiatrist will be available to answer questions in case of emergencies. Careful attention to the patient's fears and wishes with regard to his or her treatment is essential in establishing and maintaining the therapeutic alliance. Management of the therapeutic alliance should include an awareness of transference and countertransference phenomena and requires sensitive management by the psychiatrist, even if not directly addressed.

5. Monitoring the patient's psychiatric status

As treatment progresses, the different elements of panic disorder often resolve at different points. Usually, panic attacks are controlled first, but subthreshold panic attacks may linger and require further treatment. The fear that attacks may occur in the future often continues even after the attacks themselves appear to have ceased. The psychiatrist should continue to monitor the status of all of the symptoms with which the patient originally presented and should monitor the success of the treatment plan on an ongoing basis.

Finally, many illnesses, including depression and substance use disorders, co-occur with panic disorder at higher rates than are seen in the general population. Depression can develop even during successful treatment of panic disorder. Failure to recognize an emergent depression can seriously compromise therapeutic outcome.

6. Providing education to the patient and, when appropriate, to the family

Many patients with panic disorder believe they are suffering from a disorder of an organ system other than the central nervous system. They may fervently believe they have heart or lung disease. On the other hand, the significant others of patients with panic disorder frequently insist that absolutely nothing is wrong with the patient, using as evidence the fact that extensive medical testing has yielded unremarkable results (16). Under these circumstances, the patient becomes demoralized and isolated while the family can become angry or rejecting. Educating both the family and the patient and emphasizing that panic disorder is a real illness requiring support and treatment can be critical in some situations. Regardless of the method of treatment selected, successful therapies of panic disorder usually begin by explaining to the patient that the attacks themselves are not life threatening; the family may be helped to understand that panic attacks are terrifying to the patient and that the disorder, unless treated, is debilitating.

7. Working with other physicians

Patients with panic disorder often have long-standing relationships with other physicians. Because the patient is often convinced that the panic attacks represent serious abnormalities of other organ systems, a variety of general medical physicians may be involved. Psychiatric management usually requires two approaches in such cases. First, the psychiatrist may be called on to educate nonpsychiatric physicians about the ability of panic attacks to masquerade as many other general medical conditions. Although a general medical evaluation is necessary to rule out important treatable general medical conditions, there is usually little to be gained from extensive medical testing. Attempting to diagnose and treat a variety of nonspecific medical complaints sometimes only delays initiation of treatment of the panic disorder itself. Second, nonpsychiatric physicians can become frustrated with patients with panic disorder. The psychiatrist may need to intervene to ensure that the patient with panic disorder continues to receive an appropriate level of medical care from the primary care physician and medical specialists.

8. Enhancing treatment compliance

The treatment of panic disorder involves confronting many things that the patient fears. Patients are often afraid of medically adverse events; hence, they fear taking medication and are very sensitive to all somatic sensations induced by them. Some psychotherapies require the patient to confront phobic situations and often to keep careful records of anxious thoughts. These can also cause an initial increase in anxiety for the patient. The anxiety produced by treatment may lead to noncompliance. Patients stop taking medication abruptly or fail to complete required assignments during behavioral therapy. Recognition of this possibility guides the physician to design an approach to treatment that encourages the patient to articulate his or her fears. The treatment must be conducted in a completely supportive environment so that missed sessions and lapses in taking medication or carrying out behavioral and cognitive tasks are understood as part of the illness or as manifestations of issues in the therapist-patient relationship.

Family members may play a helpful role in improving treatment compliance. If compliance is not improved with discussion of fears, reassurance, nonpunitive acceptance, educational measures, and similar measures, it may be an indication of more complex resistance that is out of the patient's awareness and may be an indication for a psychodynamic treatment approach.

9. Working with the patient to address early signs of relapse

Studies have shown that panic disorder can be a chronic illness. Sometimes, an exacerbation of symptoms can occur even while the patient is undergoing treatment. This can be disconcerting and needs to be dealt with in two ways: by reassuring the patient that fluctuations in symptom levels can occur during treatment before an acceptable level of remission is reached and by evaluating whether changes in the treatment plan are warranted. Although treatment works for most patients to reduce the burden of panic disorder, patients may continue to have lingering symptoms, including occasional panic attacks of minor severity and residual avoidance. Depression can occur at any time. Relapse following treatment cessation is also always possible. Patients need to be instructed that panic disorder sometimes recurs and that if it does it is important to initiate treatment quickly to avoid the onset of complications such as phobic avoidance (17). The patient should know that he or she is welcome to contact the psychiatrist and that rapid reinitiation of treatment almost always results in improvement.

B. INTERPRETING RESULTS FROM STUDIES OF TREATMENTS FOR PANIC DISORDER

1. Measurement of outcomes

In the following sections the available data on the efficacy of treatments for panic disorder are reviewed. Short-term efficacy has usually been evaluated in 6–12-week clinical trials by observing the change in symptom ratings over the course of treatment. These outcome measures all assess a variety of panic and phobia symptoms, generally derived from the DSM-IV definition of panic attacks. Both the patient and the clinician can be asked to rate the presence and severity of a patient's symptoms. Patients have been designated as "panic free" if they do not have a sufficient number of panic symptoms to meet the DSM-IV criteria for panic disorder. However, patients labeled as "panic free" may not necessarily be free of all panic symptoms (i.e., symptom free). Another outcome measure that has been employed to assess short-term treatment response is the proportion of patients achieving remission (usually defined as the absence of panic attacks within a specified period of time).

The long-term efficacy of treatments has been measured in terms of relapse rates among panic-free or symptom-free patients receiving treatment over the course of several years. A variety of definitions of relapse have been used, based on the emergence of a certain number of symptoms or based on the percentage of change in scores on symptom rating scales. In some studies, requests for or use of additional treatment have been considered indicative of relapse; while such outcome measures may reflect an intervention's effect on patient functioning, as well as symptoms, they may also be affected by other clinical and nonclinical factors.

2. Issues in study design and interpretation

When evaluating clinical trials of medications for panic disorder, it is important to take into consideration whether a placebo group was used, the type of placebo, and the response rate in the placebo group. Response rates as high as 75% have been observed among patients receiving placebo in clinical trials of patients with panic disorder (18). High placebo response rates could explain much of the observed treatment effect in uncontrolled trials or make significant treatment effects more difficult to detect in controlled trials. It is also important to consider the dose of medication(s) employed in pharmacologic trials.

When evaluating studies of psychosocial treatments, such as CBT, which consist of multiple elements, it may be difficult to know which elements are responsible for producing beneficial outcomes. It is also important to consider the nature of the elements that were used. For example, although the types of CBT used in recent trials have been rigorously defined and have been similar, they have not been identical (19–21).

Another factor to consider is the use of medications that are not prescribed as part of the treatment protocol. For example, patients in studies of CBT may be using prescription medications that are not controlled for. In addition, patients in medication studies may be taking additional doses of the tested medications or other anti-panic medications (either explicitly, as doses taken as needed, or surreptitiously). Studies that monitor such occurrences have shown rates as high as 33% (22).

C. SPECIFIC PSYCHOSOCIAL INTERVENTIONS

Psychosocial interventions, such as psychotherapy, have traditionally been the predominant psychiatric treatment for patients with panic disorder. However, unlike medication therapies, it has been more difficult to clearly define aspects of psychosocial therapies, such as the elements they consist of and the "doses." Only recently have some psychosocial treatments been more formally operationalized and evaluated.

At the present time, cognitive behavioral treatments for panic disorder have been the most well studied. Other forms of psychotherapy are widely used for patients with panic disorder but have undergone less empirical testing. These treatments may be very different from cognitive behavioral interventions. One important difference is that many forms of psychotherapy focus broadly on the patient's current life and history, rather than more narrowly on panic-related symptoms.

1. Cognitive behavioral therapy

a. Goals

CBT is a symptom-oriented approach to the treatment of panic disorder. The treatments employed in recent clinical trials contain the following key components:

- psychoeducation
- continuous panic monitoring
- breathing retraining
- cognitive restructuring focused on correction of catastrophic misinterpretation of bodily sensations
- exposure to fear cues

The types of therapy encompassed by CBT are likely to be more diverse, and such diverse approaches have not been studied.

1) Psychoeducation. CBT always begins with one or more sessions for the purpose of psychoeducation. The aims of such sessions are to identify and name the patient's symptoms, provide a direct explanation of the basis for the symptoms, and outline a plan for the treatment. The initial education for patients is generally imparted in a didactic fashion. Exercises that actually evoke panic symptoms, such as hyperventilation, may be useful for illustrating the role of interoceptive (i.e., internal) cues in panic disorder.

2) Continuous panic monitoring. Patients are also instructed to continuously monitor their panic attacks and record their anxious cognitions, using techniques such as keeping a daily diary. Patients are informed that this will help in the assessment of the frequency and nature of their panic attacks and provide data regarding the relationship of panic symptoms to internal stimuli (e.g., emotions) and external stimuli (e.g., substances).

3) Breathing retraining. Next, the therapist introduces an anxiety management technique, such as abdominal breathing, to control the physiologic reactivity. The patient is asked to practice this technique daily.

4) Cognitive restructuring. These techniques are used to identify and counter fear of bodily sensations. Most commonly, such thinking involves overestimation of the probability of a negative consequence and catastrophic thinking about the meaning of such sensations. Patients are encouraged to consider the evidence and to think of alternative possible outcomes following the experience of the bodily cue. Part of this process involves identifying the likely origin of the feared sensations and/or any misinformation about the meaning of the sensations. The cognitive restructuring component of CBT is usually conducted by using a Socratic teaching method.

5) Exposure to fear cues. The final and central component of the treatment involves actual exposure to fear cues. In order to conduct such exposure, the therapist frequently works with the patient to identify a hierarchy of fear-evoking situations. The degree of anxiety elicited in each of these situations is graded on a 0–10 scale, and several situations that evoke anxiety at each level are documented. The patient is then asked to enter situations, usually at the low end of the hierarchy, on a regular (usually daily) basis until the fear has attenuated. The situation that arouses the next level of anxiety is then targeted. Employing more intense initial exposures and not proceeding in a graduated manner, referred to as "flooding," has also been used (23). Examples of exposures to panic cues are having patients run in place, spin in a desk chair, and breathe through a straw. The cues for panic attacks are generally interoceptive, while those for agoraphobia may be either interoceptive or environmental (24). Interoceptive exposures are usually conducted in the therapist's office and at home in naturalistic situations. Agoraphobic exposure is best carried out in the actual situation(s).

b. Efficacy

CBT efficacy studies have generally involved either cognitive behavioral treatment (as just described) or cognitive therapy. Studies of agoraphobia use behavioral exposure treatment (25, 26). A recent presentation of data from 26 subjects supports the efficacy of combining these approaches (27).

Twelve randomized controlled trials of CBT for panic disorder were identified and reviewed (19–21, 28–36). The length of treatment varied from 4 weeks to 16 weeks, and the number of subjects per cell varied from nine to 34. The degree of agoraphobia was none to mild in most of the studies. The control treatment was a wait list in five of these, a relaxation component alone in five, supportive psychotherapy in three, and a placebo medication in two. The results are shown in table 1. The results in the control conditions suggest that length of treatment and perhaps the specific interventions used may be important in determining efficacy. However, more data are necessary before firm conclusions can be drawn. Also of note, 38% of the patients in the eight studies for which medication data were given were taking some medications that were not specifically part of the study protocols (range, 0%–70%).

Several studies have examined the use of one component of CBT, behavioral exposure, for specifically agoraphobia symptoms in patients with panic disorder (35, 37–41). These studies support the efficacy of behavioral treatment in reducing phobic symptoms for patients who are able and willing to complete a treatment program of a few months. Patients who were virtually homebound were included in some of these studies, indicating that there is no need to reserve this treatment for milder or less chronic cases.

Long-term follow-ups of panic disorder range from 6 months to 8 years (20, 29, 33, 36–38, 42, 43). The three studies that included at least 1 year of follow-up showed promising results, with an

TABLE 1. Results of 12 randomized controlled studies of cognitive behavioral therapy for patients with panic disorder

Treatment	Response rate (%)
Cognitive behavioral therapy (12–15 weeks)	
Intent to treat	66
Completers	78
Control treatments	
Wait list	26
Relaxation only	
Intent to treat	45
Completers	56
Placebo	
Intent to treat	34
Completers	33
Supportive psychotherapy completers	
16 weeks	78
8 weeks	25
4 weeks	8

average of 88% of subjects remaining panic free. However, a closer look at the results in one study indicates that the percentage of patients who remained panic free throughout the 24-month period was only about 50%, and only 21% were panic free and had achieved "high end-state functioning" consistently throughout the follow-up period (43). "High end-state functioning" refers to a low severity of overall panic disorder symptoms, including anticipatory anxiety, limited-symptom episodes, and phobic symptoms in addition to panic attacks. These follow-up results are comparable to those found in medication treatment follow-up studies. One review of a series of studies also indicated that the improvement in agoraphobia and in disability after exposure therapy persists for 4 to 8 years (44).

c. Adverse effects

Cognitive behavioral exposure is a relatively benign type of intervention. However, exposure to feared situations does initially increase anxiety, and this could be considered an adverse effect. Sometimes the patient develops dependence on the therapist, which may need to be addressed. Another limitation of CBT is that it may not address other psychological problems that patients with panic disorder may have. While these problems may be less prominent than the panic disorder symptoms for many patients, some patients present with serious current and/or ongoing environmental stresses and/or other comorbid psychiatric disorders. For these patients, panic symptom relief may be less helpful, or even relatively unimportant, as a focus of treatment.

d. Implementation issues

1) **Patient acceptance.**   CBT requires considerable time and discipline on the part of the patient. Exercises must be practiced daily, and monitoring must be done continuously. In addition, patients must be willing to confront feared situations. Approximately 10%–30% of patients are unable or unwilling to complete these requirements (19, 29, 30, 33). The treatment is far less effective for these patients. Despite these limitations, however, data from several studies (39, 45, 46) indicate that more patients with panic disorder who seek treatment are willing to accept a nonmedication approach than medication.

2) **Group treatment.**   CBT for panic disorder is usually provided individually, in approximately 12 sessions, but there is evidence that group treatments may be equally effective (33, 47–51). Exposure treatments for patients with agoraphobia are often conducted in groups, and this approach has been used in many studies documenting efficacy. In addition, the inclusion of the spouse or significant other in agoraphobic treatment has been studied and found to enhance treatment efficacy (52). In this couples approach, the support person is included in psychoeducation sessions and is given a role as an assistant in exposure exercises.

3) Withdrawal of anxiolytics.   The discontinuation of benzodiazepines, such as alprazolam or clonazepam, for patients with panic disorder is often accompanied by withdrawal symptoms and relapse into panic disorder. Several studies have shown that using adjunctive CBT in this clinical situation results in successful discontinuation of the benzodiazepine for significantly more patients (53–55).

2. Psychodynamic psychotherapy

a. Goals

Psychodynamic psychotherapy is based on the concept that symptoms result from mental processes that may be outside of the patient's conscious awareness and that elucidating these processes can lead to remission of symptoms (56, 57). Moreover, in order to lessen vulnerability to panic, the psychodynamic therapist considers it necessary to identify and alter core conflicts (56). The goals of psychodynamic psychotherapy range considerably and may be more ambitious and require more time to achieve than those of a more symptom-focused treatment approach. There are some case reports of brief dynamic psychotherapies that took no longer than CBT to achieve reasonable treatment goals for patients with panic disorder (58–61). One recent study compared CBT to an emotion-focused brief psychotherapy and showed them to be equivalent (62). When combined with short-term symptomatic treatment, this approach may produce optimal long-term outcome for some patients.

b. Efficacy

There are no published reports of randomized controlled trials evaluating the efficacy of this approach for panic disorder. Studies documenting a role for both recent and early life events in the development of panic disorder, as well as a number of studies showing that patients with panic disorder remember the behavior and attitudes of their parents as more overprotective and less caring than do control subjects, provide indirect support for some aspects of the theory. One study documented the usefulness of psychodynamic psychotherapy as an adjunct to medication for outpatients with and without agoraphobia (63). In a second study (35), the control treatment of reflective listening produced results equivalent to those for CBT. In addition, a number of anecdotal case reports of successful psychodynamic treatment appear in the literature. Most of these are reports of isolated cases rather than systematic consecutive case series, and reliable, validated outcome measures were not used. Milrod et al. (56) have published a treatment manual for panic-focused psychodynamic psychotherapy, and a pilot test of outcome and of the ability of trained psychoanalysts to follow this manual is currently under way. An ongoing randomized controlled trial uses a manualized psychodynamically informed approach called "emotion-focused treatment." However, this treatment also contains cognitive, behavioral, and experiential components and differs substantially from the treatment described by Milrod et al.

c. Adverse effects

In general, psychodynamic psychotherapy has relatively few side effects. As with any psychotherapy, psychological dependency must be skillfully managed so as to facilitate treatment rather than prolong it unduly.

d. Implementation issues

In psychodynamic psychotherapy, the successful emotional and cognitive understanding of the various elements of psychic conflict (impulses, conscience and internal standards that are often excessively harsh, psychological defensive patterns, and realistic concerns) and reintegration of these elements in a more realistic and adaptive way may result in symptom resolution and fewer relapses. To achieve this insight and acceptance, the therapist places the symptoms in the context of the patient's life history and current realities and extensively uses the therapeutic relationship to focus on unconscious symptom determinants.

There are a variety of methods for conducting dynamic psychotherapy (64). Generally, the clinical approach of dynamic psychiatrists is less directive than that of behavioral therapists or psychopharmacologists. In a psychodynamic psychotherapy, it is important to consider the risks and benefits of substituting the therapist's executive functions for those of the patient. Transference considerations and the patient's freedom to associate into unexpected material must be taken into account. Some CBT techniques can be combined with psychodynamic techniques (56, 65). Clinically, as with other treatment approaches, patient factors are important determinants of the length and intensity of appropriate treatment and of specific interventions the psychiatrist may employ.

3. Combined treatments

Investigators have examined use of the combination of medication and CBT for patients with panic disorder and agoraphobia. Several short-term treatment studies have shown that the combination of the TCA imipramine with one component of CBT, behavioral exposure, may be superior to either treatment alone (66–72). Another study showed that the SSRI paroxetine plus cognitive therapy worked significantly better for patients with panic disorder than cognitive therapy plus placebo (73).

There has been one study of the combination of psychodynamic psychotherapy with medication (63). This study suggested that psychodynamic psychotherapy may improve the long-term outcome of medication-treated patients.

4. Group therapy

Reports in the literature of group therapy in the treatment of panic disorder have consisted primarily of cognitive behavioral approaches. Telch et al. (33) found a greater proportion of panic-free subjects among those who had been given group CBT than among delayed-treatment control subjects (85% versus 30%); the authors concluded that the improvements with group CBT were comparable to those in studies of individually administered CBT and pharmacologic treatment. Fifteen patients who had incomplete responses to pharmacotherapy were treated by Pollack et al. (74) with 12 weeks of group CBT and had subsequent improvements in the number of panic attacks and in scores on the Clinical Global Impression. CBT was also used concurrently with medication in a group setting for acute treatment of panic disorder (75).

Mindfulness meditation is an additional treatment proposed for panic disorder (76). This treatment is administered in a group format and includes an attention-focusing component and relaxation strategies. In one study, an 8-week trial of mindfulness meditation resulted in significant reductions in ratings of anxiety symptoms and panic attacks (77). However, it has not been compared to other, proven treatments. A 3-year follow-up showed continued beneficial effects. Other types of groups, such as medication support groups and consumer-run self-help groups, can also provide useful adjunctive experiences for patients with panic disorder.

5. Marital and family therapy

Some of the earliest theories of agoraphobia postulated an interpersonal basis for the symptoms, and some researchers have investigated the possibility that the results of behavioral treatment of agoraphobia can be enhanced by treatment of the couple or family system. While the issue has not been studied directly, patients with panic disorder without agoraphobia have symptoms that can disrupt day-to-day patterns of relationships and may place a family member in a caretaker or rescuer role. Increased dependency needs of patients with panic disorder may lead to frustration in family members, and relationships may be jeopardized. Empirical studies of the quality of marital relationships have provided mixed results; some investigators have reported that patients with agoraphobia and their spouses are not different from happily married couples (78, 79), while others show problems (80). Several studies have documented increased marital distress in some patients following successful treatment for agoraphobia (81, 82), although in general these investigators found treatment to improve marital satisfaction. In summary, there seems to be a subgroup of these patients who experience marital and/or other family distress and may benefit from a family intervention (83).

There is no published research on the use of marital or family therapy alone or with medication for the treatment of panic or agoraphobia, so no conclusions can be drawn about the potential efficacy of such an approach. Education of family members about the nature of the illness and inclusion of the spouse in the treatment may be helpful. There is a small literature exploring the benefits of including the spouse in treatment. Overall, it is clear that such a strategy is not detrimental, and results are mixed as to whether it helps. Two studies by the same research group (84, 85) show the superiority of treatment that includes the spouse as co-therapist over treatment without spouse involvement. One study (86) documented further improvement by addition of communication skills training.

6. Patient support groups

Patient support groups are very helpful for some patients suffering from panic disorder. Patients have the opportunity to learn that they are not unique in experiencing panic attacks and to share ways of coping with the illness. Support groups may also have a positive effect in encouraging patients to confront phobic situations. Finally, family members of patients with panic disorder may benefit from the educational aspects of patient support groups. In deciding to refer a patient to a support group, however, it is imperative that the psychiatrist obtain information about the nature of the group and the credentials of its leader(s). Support groups are not a substitute for effective treatment; rather, they are complementary.

D. PHARMACOLOGIC INTERVENTIONS

Medications have been known to be useful in the treatment of panic disorder for over 30 years. Most studies have focused on their ability to stop or reduce the frequency of panic attacks, but many have also addressed the effect of medication on anticipatory anxiety, phobic avoidance, associated depression, and global function. Medications from several classes have been shown to be effective. As discussed in section III.B, when interpreting results from trials of pharmacologic interventions, it is important to consider whether a placebo group was used and the response rate in the placebo group.

1. Selective serotonin reuptake inhibitors

a. Goals

The primary goals of SSRI therapy of panic disorder are to reduce the intensity and frequency of panic attacks, to reduce anticipatory anxiety, and to treat associated depression. Often, successful therapy with SSRIs also leads to a reduction in phobic avoidance.

b. Efficacy

Four SSRIs are now available in the United States: fluoxetine, sertraline, paroxetine, and fluvoxamine. Clinical trials indicating that each of them is effective for panic disorder have now been completed.

Results of one multicenter double-blind, randomized trial that compared two doses of fluoxetine (10 mg/day and 20 mg/day) with placebo have been presented (87). Reductions in panic symptoms, measured by using several instruments, were significantly greater for patients treated with 20 mg/day of fluoxetine than those given placebo. Fluoxetine at 10 mg/day showed superiority over placebo for only a few assessments of panic symptoms. Two open studies of fluoxetine treatment for panic disorder have been published. Gorman et al. (88) found that of 16 patients whose fluoxetine dose began at 10 mg/day and was raised in 10 mg/day increments each week, only 44% eventually responded to fluoxetine (mean dose among responders was 27.1 mg/day); however, 90% of the nonresponders had been unable to tolerate the side effects. Schneier et al. (89), initiating fluoxetine treatment at 5 mg/day and using a more conservative titration schedule with 25 patients, found that 76%

had moderate to marked improvements (median dose among responders was 20 mg/day).

Results from two multicenter randomized, double-blind, placebo-controlled trials of sertraline have been presented at recent public meetings but had not been published by 1996. Wolkow et al. (90) reported that patients treated with sertraline had a significantly greater reduction in panic attack frequency than those given placebo (79% versus 59% reduction). Similarly, Baumel et al. (91) found a significantly greater reduction in panic attack frequency for patients given sertraline than for those given placebo (77% versus 51% reduction).

Paroxetine, which has received approval from the U.S. Food and Drug Administration (FDA) for treatment of panic disorder, has been studied in several placebo-controlled trials. One double-blind trial compared paroxetine plus cognitive therapy to placebo plus cognitive therapy; significantly more patients in the paroxetine group (82% versus 50%) achieved a 50% reduction in panic attack frequency (73). Ballenger et al. (92) compared placebo to three doses of paroxetine; the percentages of patients given paroxetine at daily doses of 40 mg, 20 mg, and 10 mg and patients given placebo who were subsequently panic free were 86%, 65%, 67%, and 50%, respectively (only the difference between 40-mg paroxetine and placebo was statistically significant). In another double-blind trial (93), 367 patients were randomly assigned to paroxetine, clomipramine, or placebo. Paroxetine (at a mean final dose of 39 mg/day) was found to be superior to placebo and comparable to clomipramine (mean final dose of 92 mg/day).

Several controlled trials of fluvoxamine for panic disorder have also been published. In one (94), more patients who had been given fluvoxamine than placebo were panic free (61% versus 36%). Black et al. (32) compared fluvoxamine to a modified form of cognitive therapy and to placebo; there were more panic-free patients in the fluvoxamine group (81%) than in either the cognitive therapy (50%) or placebo (39%) group (only the difference between fluvoxamine and placebo was significant). In other studies fluvoxamine has proved to be better than maprotiline and an experimental serotonin-blocking medication, ritanserin (95, 96). Citalopram, an SSRI available in Europe, was studied in one double-blind trial in which 475 patients were randomly assigned to citalopram (10–15 mg/day, 20–30 mg/day, or 40–60 mg/day), clomipramine (60–90 mg/day), or placebo (97). Citalopram at 20–30 or 40–60 mg/day was significantly superior to placebo; citalopram at 20–30 mg/day was more effective than 40–60 mg/day and comparable to clomipramine.

Although the database for SSRI therapy of panic disorder is not yet as extensive as that for either imipramine or alprazolam, there are sufficient controlled trials available to state that these medications have demonstrated short-term efficacy in treating panic attacks. A meta-analysis (98) of 27 studies involving 2,348 patients in randomized, prospective, double-blind, placebo-controlled trials suggested that the effect size for improvement with SSRIs in panic disorder is significantly greater than for alprazolam or imipramine.

c. Side effects

SSRIs are safer than TCAs. They are not lethal in overdose and have few serious effects on cardiovascular function. Because they lack clinically significant anticholinergic effects, they can be prescribed to patients with prostatic hypertrophy or narrow-angle glaucoma. Because elimination of SSRIs involves hepatic metabolism, doses need to be adjusted for patients with liver disease and dysfunction.

The main side effects of SSRIs are headaches, irritability, nausea and other gastrointestinal complaints, insomnia, sexual dysfunctions, increased anxiety, drowsiness, and tremor. There are scattered reports in the literature of extrapyramidal side effects, but these have not been observed in large multicenter trials and may be idiosyncratic. There is no evidence that SSRIs increase suicidal or violent behavior.

There are a number of published case reports of a withdrawal syndrome caused by the abrupt discontinuation of SSRIs (99). Black et al. (32) abruptly withdrew fluvoxamine from patients with panic disorder after 8 months of treatment. A withdrawal syndrome characterized by dizziness, incoordination, headache, irritability, and nausea began within 24 hours, peaked at day 5 after withdrawal, and was generally resolved by day 14.

d. Implementation issues

1) **Dose.** As is the case with tricyclics, some patients with panic disorder experience an initial feeling of increased anxiety, jitteriness, shakiness, and agitation when beginning treatment with an SSRI. For that reason, the initial dose should be lower than that usually prescribed to patients with depression. Louie et al. (100), for example, found that patients with both panic disorder and major depression were less tolerant of higher doses of fluoxetine than patients with major depression alone. The recommended starting doses for SSRIs are as follows: fluoxetine, 10 mg/day or less; sertraline, 25 mg/day; paroxetine, 10 mg/day; and fluvoxamine, 50 mg/day. In the few published studies, fluoxetine has been found to be effective at doses ranging between 5 and 80 mg/day. Recent case reports suggest that for some patients fluoxetine taken in doses as low as 1–2 mg/day may be effective (101). For paroxetine, in a clinical trial the lowest dose that was significantly superior to placebo was 40 mg/day, although some patients did respond to lower doses (92). For sertraline, a fixed-dose study suggests that doses of 50, 100, and 200 mg/day are equally effective for panic disorder (102). Fluvoxamine has been found effective in doses up to 300 mg/day. It is recommended that the initial low dose of the SSRI be maintained for several days and then increased to a more standard daily dose (e.g., 20 mg of fluoxetine or paroxetine, 50 mg of sertraline, 150 mg of fluvoxamine). Patients who fail to respond after several weeks may then do better with a further dose increase.

2) **Length of treatment.** Studies of SSRI therapy for panic disorder have been conducted over 6 to 12 weeks and even longer

periods. It is generally accepted that response does not occur for at least 4 weeks, and some patients will not realize full response for 8 to 12 weeks.

There are few data on the optimum length of treatment following response. Gergel et al. (103) selected patients who had responded to paroxetine in an acute-phase trial and randomly assigned them to placebo or 10, 20, or 40 mg/day of paroxetine for a 12-week maintenance period. After the maintenance phase, there was a significantly higher rate of relapse among the responders who had crossed over to placebo than those whose paroxetine treatment had been maintained (30% versus 5%).

LeCrubier et al. (93) evaluated the efficacy of paroxetine, clomipramine, and placebo for patients who completed a 12-week double-blind trial and then chose to continue receiving the randomly assigned treatment for an additional 36 weeks. Compared with the placebo-treated patients, the paroxetine patients experienced significantly greater reductions in panic symptoms, and a larger proportion remained free of panic attacks throughout the long-term study. There were no significant differences in efficacy between paroxetine and clomipramine.

If the medications are to be discontinued after prolonged use, it is recommended that the SSRI dose be tapered over several weeks. It is not clear whether this is necessary for fluoxetine, which has the longest half-life of any medication in the class.

2. Tricyclic antidepressants

a. Goals

The primary goals of TCA therapy of panic disorder are to reduce the intensity and frequency of panic attacks, to reduce anticipatory anxiety, and to treat associated depression. Successful tricyclic therapy also leads to a reduction in phobic avoidance.

b. Efficacy

The first controlled study documenting the efficacy of the tricyclic imipramine in blocking panic attacks was conducted by Klein and published in 1964 (104). In this study, imipramine was superior to placebo for antipanic effect and for change in the Clinical Global Impression (CGI). Since then, 15 controlled trials (16, 66, 105–117) have shown that imipramine is effective in reducing panic. After treatment with imipramine, 45%–70% of the patients were found to be panic free, compared to 15%–50% of those receiving placebo. In addition, patients with panic disorder who were treated with imipramine had less phobic avoidance and anticipatory anxiety than those receiving placebo. Typically, patients treated with imipramine realize a substantial reduction in panic after a minimum of 4 weeks of treatment; antipanic effect may not be fully experienced until 8 to 12 weeks of therapy. Anticipatory anxiety usually responds after the panic attacks have been reduced, and phobic avoidance is the last to be affected.

Given the equivalency of tricyclic agents in treating depression, there is little reason to expect tricyclics other than imipramine to work less well for panic disorder. However, very few controlled studies have evaluated other tricyclics for panic disorder. Lydiard et al. (18) found desipramine to be superior to placebo for a global measure of phobic avoidance and score on the Hamilton Rating Scale for Anxiety, but there was only a trend toward superiority (p<0.09) on the CGI. Although 85% of the desipramine-treated patients had reductions in panic attacks, this was not significantly different from the 76% for the placebo-treated patients. One double-blind comparative study showed the tricyclic maprotiline to be less effective than the SSRI fluvoxamine (118).

Two studies have shown that clomipramine is at least as effective as imipramine. There are anecdotal reports that clomipramine is actually somewhat more effective than imipramine; however, the evidence from the few studies that have directly compared the two is equivocal. In one double-blind, placebo-controlled study (106), clomipramine (mean dose, 109 mg/day) was superior to both imipramine (mean dose, 124 mg/day) and placebo in panic reduction and decrease in score on the Hamilton anxiety scale. In a nonblind, uncontrolled trial, Cassano et al. (119) did not find significant differences between clomipramine (mean dose, 128 mg/day) and imipramine (mean dose, 144 mg/day).

c. Side effects

The major adverse side effects common to all tricyclic medications and reported in studies of panic disorder treatment are 1) anticholinergic: dry mouth, constipation, difficulty urinating, increased heart rate, and blurry vision; 2) increased sweating; 3) sleep disturbance; 4) orthostatic hypotension and dizziness; 5) fatigue and weakness; 6) cognitive disturbance; 7) weight gain, especially for long-term users; and 8) sexual dysfunction (120). Higher doses are associated with a higher dropout rate in research studies. For example, Mavissakalian and Perel (110) reported that among subjects treated with an average of 35, 99, and 200 mg/day of imipramine, the dropout rates due to drug side effects were 6%, 15%, and 36%, respectively. TCAs should not be prescribed for patients with panic disorder who also have acute narrow-angle glaucoma or clinically significant prostatic hypertrophy. Patients with cardiac conduction abnormalities may experience a severe or fatal arrhythmia with tricyclics. Overdoses with TCAs can lead to significant cardiac toxicity and fatality; for this reason, TCAs may be suboptimal for suicidal patients. Elderly patients may be at increased risk of falls because of orthostatic hypotension caused by tricyclics.

d. Implementation issues

1) Dose. Clinicians have often noticed, and research studies have occasionally shown, that some patients with panic disorder are exquisitely sensitive to both the beneficial and adverse effects of tricyclics. Zitrin et al. (66) found that 20% of the patients in their study could not tolerate doses higher than 10 mg/day but still experienced panic blockade. Lydiard et al. (18) also reported an initial supersensitivity in some patients with panic disorder. Patients sometimes experience a stimulant-like response, including anxiety, agitation, or insomnia, when treatment with antidepressant medication of any class is initiated. For this reason, it is recommended that tricyclics be started for patients with panic disorder at doses substantially lower than those for patients with depression or other psychiatric conditions. One common strategy is to begin with only 10 mg/day of imipramine and gradually titrate the dose upward over the ensuing weeks.

Few studies have rigorously addressed the optimum dose of tricyclic medication for panic disorder. In most research studies, the mean final dose is approximately 150 mg/day and the maximum final dose is up to 300 mg/day. Mavissakalian and Perel (110) randomly assigned patients with panic disorder to low-dose (mean, 35 mg/day), medium-dose (mean, 99 mg/day), and high-dose (mean, 200 mg/day) imipramine. They found that both the medium and high doses were superior to placebo in reducing panic and not significantly different from each other; the low dose was no more effective than placebo. Given these findings, it is reasonable to titrate the imipramine dose of patients with panic disorder to approximately 100 mg/day and wait for at least 4 weeks to see whether there is a response. If tolerated, the dose can then be increased to as high as 300 mg/day if initial response is either absent or inadequate.

There is a suggestion in the literature that clomipramine may be effective in somewhat lower doses than imipramine. Clomipramine can generally be used effectively with doses less than 150 mg/day. Given the results of the studies by Modigh et al. (106) and Cassano et al. (119), it may be reasonable to administer clomipramine in a dose range of 25–150 mg/day.

2) Length of treatment.   Most controlled trials of tricyclics for the treatment of panic disorder were for a minimum of 8 weeks, and exactly when the patients began to respond has not always been reported. There is general clinical agreement that, similar to the situation with treatment of depression, it may take at least 4 weeks of tricyclic treatment for onset of antipanic effects; patients may not respond until 6 or even 8 weeks, and some additional response has been seen through 12 or more weeks. It is reasonable to wait for at least 6 weeks from initiation of tricyclic treatment, with at least 2 of those weeks at full dose, before deciding whether a tricyclic is effective for a patient with panic disorder. If there is some response at this point, the clinician and patient may wait longer to see how full the response will be by 8 to 12 weeks.

There are few long-term studies of tricyclic treatment for panic disorder in the literature. Cassano et al. (112) continued to treat patients with imipramine or placebo for 6 months after an acute-phase 8-week study and found that imipramine was still superior to placebo for panic reduction. Curtis et al. (113) also maintained patients on a regimen of placebo or imipramine for up to 8 months after acute 8-week treatment and found that the placebo-treated patients had more panic attacks and phobic avoidance and were more likely to drop out of treatment during the maintenance phase. In two small studies, Mavissakalian and Perel (121, 122) assessed the relapse rates of patients nonrandomly assigned to either a) discontinuation of imipramine following 6 months of full-dose imipramine plus 1 year of half-dose imipramine maintenance treatment or b) discontinuation following 6 months of acute imipramine treatment alone. They found significantly less relapse among the patients who had been in treatment for 18 months than among those who had been treated for 6 months. These studies suggest that maintenance treatment is beneficial for at least a year after a patient has achieved a response to a tricyclic. The exact relapse rate following discontinuation of imipramine or other tricyclic therapy is also not known (123, 124).

3. Benzodiazepines

a. Goals

The primary goals of benzodiazepine therapy of panic disorder are to reducc the intensity and frequency of panic attacks and to reduce anticipatory anxiety. Often, successful benzodiazepine therapy also leads to a reduction in phobic avoidance.

b. Efficacy

Alprazolam has been studied more extensively than any other benzodiazepine for the treatment of panic disorder and is approved by the FDA for the treatment of panic disorder. Eleven trials of alprazolam treatment of panic disorder were reviewed, including the Cross-National Collaborative Panic Study, which involved more than 1,000 patients randomly assigned to imipramine, alprazolam, or placebo (125). Nine of the trials were double blind, and seven were placebo controlled. Two meta-analyses of studies on alprazolam treatment for panic disorder were also reviewed.

In six of the seven double-blind, placebo-controlled trials, alprazolam was found to be superior to placebo in the treatment of panic attacks (113, 126–130), while the other one did not assess panic attacks as an outcome measure (131). The percentages of patients who were panic free (generally assessed over a 1-week period) at end point were 55%–75% for alprazolam (at doses of 5–6 mg/day) and 15%–50% for placebo. These percentages represent the "intention to treat" proportions (i.e., the panic-free proportion of the patients who were originally assigned to receive active treatment or placebo at the start of the trial); the differences between the completers were less striking or nonsignificant because of higher dropout rates for the nonresponders in the placebo groups. Alprazolam was superior to placebo in reducing phobic avoidance in five of the six studies in which it was assessed, disability in five of five studies, anticipatory anxiety in three of three studies, and Hamilton anxiety scale scores in six of seven studies. In most of the studies, patients with primary current major depression were excluded and the level of phobic avoidance was moderate.

Four of the 11 trials compared alprazolam to imipramine. Three of these were double blind. Alprazolam and imipramine were comparable in efficacy for panic attacks, phobias, Hamilton anxiety scores, disability, and CGI ratings. There were more dropouts in the imipramine group in three of the four studies.

These data support the efficacy of alprazolam (especially in the 5–6 mg/day range) in treating multiple dimensions of illness in patients with panic disorder who do not have primary current major depression.

Twelve studies regarding other benzodiazepines were also reviewed (126, 128, 132–141), and they support the short-term efficacy of other benzodiazepines for panic disorder. The agents studied include clonazepam (effective in the one double-blind, placebo-controlled trial), diazepam (effective in two of two trials, both double blind and one placebo controlled), and lorazepam (equivalent to alprazolam in three of three double-blind trials). One study showed superiority of imipramine over chlordiazepoxide.

These studies suggest that other benzodiazepines (at least diazepam, clonazepam, and lorazepam), when given in equivalent doses, may be as effective as alprazolam in the treatment of panic disorder.

There was one controlled trial of alprazolam as an adjunct to imipramine for the first 4 to 6 weeks of treatment (115). The subjects taking alprazolam showed a more rapid therapeutic response, but this was not associated with a lower percentage of treatment dropout. In addition, 10 of 17 patients taking alprazolam were unable to taper from 1.5 mg/day to discontinuation in 2 weeks after 4 to 6 weeks of treatment.

c. Side effects

The adverse effects of benzodiazepines in patients with panic disorder appear similar to those reported when benzodiazepines are used for other indications and include primarily sedation, fatigue, ataxia, slurred speech, memory impairment, and weakness. Some sedation or drowsiness occurred in 38%–75% of alprazolam-treated subjects and 11%–21% of those taking placebo. Memory problems were reported by up to 15% of patients taking alprazolam and 8.5% of patients taking placebo in the Cross-National Collaborative Panic Study. However, patients may not recognize their own cognitive impairment. It is prudent to be cautious about prescribing benzodiazepines to elderly patients or those with pretreatment cognitive impairment. The risk of falls for the elderly and the increased risk of motor vehicle accidents related to benzodiazepine use should also be considered. Among patients with histories of substance abuse or dependence, benzodiazepine use may aggravate symptoms and should be avoided. In general, however, benzodiazepines seem to be well tolerated in patients with panic disorder with very few serious side effects.

Major concerns about benzodiazepine tolerance and withdrawal have been raised. According to the report of the APA Task Force on Benzodiazepine Dependence, Toxicity, and Abuse, "There are no data to suggest that long-term therapeutic use of benzodiazepines by patients commonly leads to dose escalation or to recreational abuse" (142). However, benzodiazepines may still be underused because of an inappropriate fear of addiction. The studies of long-term alprazolam treatment for panic disorder show that the doses patients use at 32 weeks of treatment are similar to those used at 8 weeks, indicating that, as a group, patients with panic disorder do not escalate alprazolam doses or display tolerance to alprazolam's therapeutic effects, at least in the first 8 months of treatment. However, studies of dose escalation following longer periods of benzodiazepine use are generally lacking.

Six studies regarding discontinuation of alprazolam for patients with panic disorder were reviewed. These studies demonstrated that significant numbers of these patients (ranging from 33% to 100%) are unable to complete a taper of the medication after 6 weeks to 22 months of treatment. One study (143) showed that alprazolam causes significantly more withdrawal symptoms, recurrent panic attacks, and failure to complete the taper than imipramine, and another (144) suggested that patients with panic disorder have more difficulty during tapering of alprazolam than do those with generalized anxiety disorder, even when the patients in both groups are treated with similar doses. Difficulties during taper seem most severe during the last half of the taper period and the first week after the taper is completed. In many instances, it is difficult to determine the extent to which symptoms are due to withdrawal, rebound, or relapse.

The one study comparing diazepam to alprazolam for panic disorder indicated that both are no different from placebo during gradual tapering of the first half of the dose (145). With abrupt discontinuation of the remaining dose, however, alprazolam caused significantly more anxiety, relapse, and rebound. In general, apart from this one study, the issue of discontinuation of benzodiazepines with short versus long half-lives or high versus low potency has not been adequately addressed in relation to panic disorder. The APA task force report on benzodiazepines (142) suggests that there are more difficulties with short-half-life, high-potency compounds. However, studies by Schweizer, Rickels, Weiss, and Zavodnick (129, 143) of benzodiazepine-treated patients showed no significant effect of half-life on the results of a gradual taper but greater withdrawal severity after abrupt discontinuation with compounds having shorter half-lives and with higher daily doses. These studies, although not involving patients with panic disorder specifically, suggest that half-life is less of a factor, or in fact may not be important, given a gradual taper schedule.

Thus, there is no evidence for significant dose escalation in patients with panic disorder (75). However, withdrawal symptoms and symptomatic rebound are commonly seen with discontinuation of alprazolam after as little as 6 to 8 weeks of treatment. These discontinuation effects appear more severe than those following taper of imipramine and may be more severe in patients with panic disorder than in those with generalized anxiety disorder. This would argue for tapering benzodiazepines very slowly for patients with panic disorder, probably over 2–4 months and at rates no higher than 10% of the dose per week (2, 146). Withdrawal symptoms can occur throughout the taper and may be especially severe toward the end of the taper. The decision of when to attempt a benzodiazepine taper may be influenced by factors such as the presence of psychosocial stressors or supports, the stability of comorbid conditions, and the availability of alternative treatment options.

d. Implementation issues

1) Dose. The manufacturer's recommendation for alprazolam treatment of panic disorder notes that doses above 4 mg/day are usually necessary and that doses up to 10 mg/day are sometimes required. However, very few studies have empirically evaluated dose requirements. Two studies (22, 105) compared alprazolam doses of 6 mg/day and 2 mg/day. The study by Uhlenhuth et al. (105) showed a significant advantage for the higher dose in producing a panic-free state. The study by Lydiard et al. (22) showed very little difference between the higher and lower doses (absence of panic attacks at study end in 65% of patients taking higher dose, 50% taking lower dose, but only 15% taking placebo). However, the rates of surreptitious benzodiazepine use for the lower-dose (23%) and placebo (35%) patients were considerably greater than the rate for the patients taking the higher alprazolam dose (4%), perhaps suggesting that the patients did not find the lower dose or placebo clinically effective. Lydiard and colleagues found that adverse side effects were more pronounced at the higher dose than at the lower dose of alprazolam. Given these findings, it is necessary to be flexible in choosing the alprazolam dose for an individual patient. Most patients require three to four doses per day to avoid breakthrough or rebound symptoms, although some may achieve symptom control with two doses of alprazolam per day. The dose should be titrated up to 2–3 mg/day at first, but an increase to 5–6 mg/day will be necessary for some patients.

In one multicenter dose-ranging trial (147), patients with panic disorder were randomly assigned to placebo or one of five fixed doses (0.5, 1.0, 2.0, 3.0, or 4.0 mg/day) of clonazepam. During 6 weeks of treatment, the minimum effective dose was 1.0 mg/day, and daily doses of 1.0 mg/day and higher were equally effective in reducing the number of panic attacks. The investigators concluded that daily doses of 1.0 to 2.0 mg of clonazepam offered the best balance of therapeutic benefits and side effects. Because of its relatively long half-life, clonazepam can usually be administered once or twice a day.

The dosing of other benzodiazepines in the treatment of panic disorder is less well established. In controlled studies, lorazepam has been given at doses of about 7 mg/day, usually two or three times daily. Diazepam doses ranged from 5 to 40 mg/day in two published trials.

Results of several studies suggest a relationship between alprazolam blood levels and treatment response (148, 149). Monitoring blood levels of alprazolam may be useful for dose adjustment, although this is not routinely done.

2) Length of treatment. Alprazolam had an earlier onset of action than imipramine in three controlled trials. Clinicians and patients often note some reduction in panic within the first week of treatment, although full blockade of panic attacks can take several weeks.

As with TCA treatment of panic disorder, there are very few data indicating the optimum length of maintenance therapy for responders to benzodiazepines. Two published trials have compared maintenance imipramine, alprazolam, and placebo treatment, and both suggest that imipramine may be superior. In the study by Cassano et al. (112), imipramine and alprazolam patients fared equally well in terms of panic reduction during a 6-month maintenance phase, but the imipramine-treated patients had less phobic avoidance. There were more alprazolam dropouts during the maintenance phase than during the 8-week acute treatment phase, while the number of imipramine dropouts did not differ between the two phases. Curtis et al. (113) found that from month 4 through the end of an 8-month maintenance phase patients taking imipramine had virtually no panic attacks, while alprazolam-treated patients continued to experience infrequent panic attacks. On all other measures, however, the two medications performed equally well. In a third investigation, by Lepola et al. (150), patients who had been treated with alprazolam (N=27) and imipramine (N=28) in a 9-week trial were then followed for 3 years in a naturalistic study. Significantly more alprazolam users than imipramine users were found to be still using their original medication after 3 years (74% versus 32%). The authors pointed out that it is difficult to know whether this difference is attributable to a better long-term response among the imipramine users than among the alprazolam users, a greater degree of intolerable side effects for the imipramine users, or greater difficulty in discontinuing treatment among the alprazolam users due to physiologic dependence.

4. Monoamine oxidase inhibitors

a. Goals

The primary goals of MAOI therapy of panic disorder are to reduce the intensity and frequency of panic attacks, to reduce anticipatory anxiety, and to treat associated depression. Often, successful therapy with MAOIs also leads to a reduction in phobic avoidance.

b. Efficacy

There have been virtually no studies involving the use of MAOIs since the introduction of the panic disorder diagnosis in DSM-III in 1980. It is therefore nearly impossible to cite controlled trials in which MAOIs that are approved for use in the United States and currently manufactured (i.e., phenelzine and tranylcypromine) have been used for the specific treatment of panic disorder with or without agoraphobia. Even the most modern and rigorous study (151) involved the use of phenelzine for the treatment of "phobic neurosis" (152). The commonly held belief that MAOIs are actually more potent antipanic agents than tricyclics has never been convincingly proven in the scientific literature and is only supported by clinical anecdote.

Two studies have looked at the effectiveness of a reversible inhibitor of monoamine oxidase A (RIMA) for panic disorder. No medication in the RIMA class is currently approved for use in the United States, but at least one, moclobemide, is widely used in Europe and Canada. These medications do not generally require adherence to the tyramine-free diet that is mandatory for patients treated with phenelzine or tranylcypromine. Both studies, one a double-blind comparison of brofaromine to clomipramine (153) and the other an open study of brofaromine (154), showed antipanic and antiphobic efficacy.

c. Side effects

Adverse side effects are clearly a major concern with MAOI therapy. The complexity of these medications suggests that they should be prescribed by physicians with experience in monitoring MAOI treatment.

The main risk of taking an MAOI is hypertensive crisis secondary to ingestion of tyramine. Hence, patients taking phenelzine or tranylcypromine must adhere to the special low-tyramine diet. Certain medications, including but not limited to sympathomimetic amines, decongestants, the over-the-counter medication dextromethorphan, and meperidine, must not be used with MAOIs. Another serious drug-drug interaction to be avoided is the "serotonergic syndrome" that can occur from the use of MAOIs with SSRIs (155). Even when the risk of hypertensive crisis is obviated by strict adherence to dietary and medication restrictions, MAOIs have substantial adverse effects. These include hypotension (sometimes leading to syncope), weight gain, hypomania, sexual dysfunction, paresthesia, sleep disturbance, myoclonic jerks, dry mouth, and edema.

d. Implementation issues

1) **Dose.**   Doses of phenelzine in controlled trials for panic-disorder-like illnesses have tended to be low, often no higher than 45 mg/day. Some authors have commented that higher doses may be more effective. Doses of phenelzine up to 90 mg/day and of tranylcypromine up to 70 mg/day are said by experienced clinicians to be necessary for some patients with panic disorder.

2) **Length of treatment.**   The onset of the antipanic effect of MAOIs generally follows the same time course as that for tricyclics. Patients rarely get significant benefit before several weeks have elapsed, and periods up to 12 weeks may be necessary before the full effectiveness of the medication can be judged.

No maintenance studies of MAOIs for panic disorder have been published. Hence, the optimal length of treatment, to provide the least chance of relapse, is not established.

5. Other antidepressants *a. Venlafaxine*

One small controlled trial at a single site, drawn from a larger multicenter trial, showed that venlafaxine (mean dose, 150 mg/day) was effective for treating panic disorder (156). A published series of four cases of patients with panic disorder indicated that venlafaxine at relatively low doses (50–75 mg/day) may be effective and well tolerated (157).

b. Trazodone

One double-blind study (158) in which 74 patients with panic disorder were assigned to trazodone, imipramine, or alprazolam showed trazodone to be less effective than either imipramine or alprazolam. However, in a single-blind study (159) in which 11 patients with panic disorder were treated with trazodone, panic symptoms improved significantly from a baseline period of placebo treatment.

c. Bupropion

Bupropion has been found to be effective in the treatment of depression. Proposed mechanisms of action include dopaminergic and noradrenergic agonist effects. Although there have been several small clinical trials using bupropion for patients with panic disorder, there is general consensus that it is not effective in alleviating either the somatic or psychological symptoms of panic attacks. It may have a role as an adjunctive treatment for patients with panic disorder who suffer sexual dysfunction as a side effect of other antidepressant medications, but it nevertheless may be potentially "overenergizing" for this specific patient group (160).

d. Nefazodone

One retrospective analysis of a randomized, placebo-controlled trial evaluated the effectiveness of nefazodone and imipramine among patients with comorbid panic disorder and major depression (161). Patients treated with nefazodone experienced significantly greater reductions in panic symptoms than placebo-treated patients; imipramine treatment was not found to be significantly better than placebo. An open-label trial examined nefazodone treatment among patients with panic disorder and concurrent depression or depressive symptoms (162). Panic symptoms were judged to be much or very much improved in 71% of the patients treated with nefazodone.

6. Anticonvulsants

There are limited data concerning the use of anticonvulsant medication in the treatment of panic disorder. In case reports, carbamazepine has been reported to improve panic attacks in patients with EEG abnormalities (163). However, the only controlled trial of carbamazepine suggested that it is not superior to placebo in reducing panic attack frequency (164). One crossover study showed significantly greater improvement in panic symptoms during periods of treatment with valproate than during treatment with placebo (165). A few reports, mostly findings from small numbers of subjects in uncontrolled studies or anecdotal reports on a few subjects, also suggest that valproate is an effective treatment for panic disorder (166). In these studies, valproate was well tolerated, but the adverse side effects included gastrointestinal dysfunction, weight gain, dizziness, nausea, sedation, and alopecia. A single case report indicated that gabapentin was effective for a patient with panic disorder.

7. Other agents

a. Conventional antipsychotic medications

Conventional antipsychotic medications are rarely appropriate in the treatment of uncomplicated panic disorder. There is no evidence that they are effective, and the risk of neurological side effects outweighs any potential benefit. There is interest, but no evidence, in the possibility that clozapine may be useful for extremely refractory cases of panic disorder. At present, however, this cannot be recommended.

b. β Blockers

The limited number of controlled trials that have been conducted with β-adrenergic blocking agents in panic disorder have provided mixed results. Noyes et al. (133) compared the efficacy of diazepam and propranolol for 21 patients with panic disorder in a double-blind crossover study. Findings revealed that 18 of the 21 patients responded "moderately" to diazepam but only seven of the 21 responded to propranolol. As the sole agent, the β blocker did not appear to be effective in alleviating phobic symptoms or panic attacks, despite adequate peripheral blockade. Munjack et al. (167) compared the effectiveness of alprazolam, propranolol, and placebo for 55 patients with panic disorder and agoraphobia. This study also showed superiority of alprazolam over propranolol: 75% of the alprazolam patients met the criterion of zero panic attacks after 5 weeks, compared with 37% of the propranolol group and 43% of the placebo patients. Ravaris et al. (168) also compared propranolol with alprazolam, but the results demonstrated that alprazolam and propranolol provided similar effects in suppressing panic attacks and reducing avoidance behaviors; the only difference in this study was the more rapid onset of action of alprazolam. One open-label, case report study (169) indicated a possible additive effect of the combination of propranolol and alprazolam. No subsequent clinical trials have addressed the issue of combination therapy with these agents.

c. Calcium channel blockers

The cardiovascular symptoms associated with panic attacks include palpitations, facial flushing, lightheadedness, paresthesia, presyncopal disturbances, and tachycardia, which have been attributed to autonomic instability. Calcium channel blockers have been used increasingly to offset these physical manifestations in anxious patients. Successful results have been achieved with regard to complaints of palpitations and hyperventilation. Calcium channel blockers have particular potential for patients with mitral valve prolapse, especially when echocardiographic data are correlated with physical manifestations of autonomic hyperactivity. Data from controlled clinical studies that delineate a specific efficacy of calcium channel blockers in panic disorder or other anxiety disorders are very limited. Klein and Uhde (170) conducted one double-blind crossover study of verapamil involving 11 patients with panic disorder. When treated with verapamil, the patients had statistically significant, although clinically modest, reductions in the number of panic attacks and severity of anxiety symptoms. Use of these agents as anxiety treatments is mostly based on empirical assumptions related to cardiovascular effects or on case study reports. More investigation is needed to determine their role in panic amelioration, whether as a first-line treatment or as an adjunctive modality.

d. Inositol

Benjamin et al. (171) reported efficacy for inositol in a small, placebo-controlled trial involving 21 patients. The dose was 12 g/day, and the side effects were reported as minimal.

e. Clonidine

Few clinical trials with clonidine for the treatment of panic disorder and other anxiety disorders have been conducted. The controlled trials that have been done were limited to relatively small groups, and the results were equivocal with regard to efficacy. Uhde et al. (172) evaluated clonidine for patients with panic disorder and noted that it was more effective than placebo in reducing anxiety as measured by the Spielberger State-Trait Anxiety Inventory (173), Zung Anxiety Scale (174), and patient reports of frequency of anxiety symptoms. Hoehn-Saric et al. (175) studied the effect of clonidine on 23 patients with generalized anxiety disorder and panic disorder. They observed that clonidine was superior to placebo in relieving psychic and somatic symptoms, but of the 14 patients with panic disorder, three worsened with this agent. Hoehn-Saric et al. also noted that clonidine was not "as good as classical anxiety agents." There was a high frequency of side effects; 95% of the patients reported undesirable effects by week 12. Results from another study indicate that if there are therapeutic effects of clonidine for patients with panic disorder, they may be transient. Uhde et al. (172) gave intravenous clonidine or placebo to patients with panic disorder and healthy control subjects. After 1 hour, they found that clonidine was significantly more effective at reducing anxiety symptoms than placebo and that patients with panic disorder had a significantly greater reduction in anxiety symptoms than the control subjects. However, among 18 patients with panic disorder given oral clonidine for an average of 10 weeks, there was no difference in anxiety symptom scores assessed before and at the end of treatment.

f. Buspirone

Buspirone has been demonstrated to be effective in the long-term treatment of psychic and somatic symptoms of generalized anxiety disorder. Thus far, however, very limited information is available regarding the efficacy of buspirone for panic disorder. Sheehan et al. (176) reported that buspirone was not superior to placebo on any outcome measure in patients with panic disorder. This study was similar in outcome to a previous study (177), which also showed that buspirone did not seem to affect the symptoms of panic disorder.

IV. DEVELOPMENT OF A TREATMENT PLAN FOR THE INDIVIDUAL PATIENT

A. CHOOSING A SITE OF TREATMENT

The treatment of panic disorder is generally conducted entirely on an outpatient basis, and the condition by itself rarely warrants hospitalization. Occasionally, the first contact between patient and psychiatrist occurs in the emergency room or the hospital when the patient has been admitted in the midst of an acute panic episode. The patient may even be admitted by emergency room staff to rule out myocardial infarction or other serious general medical events. In such cases, the psychiatrist may be able to make the diagnosis of panic disorder and initiate treatment once other general medical conditions have been ruled out. Because panic disorder is frequently comorbid with depression and appears to elevate the risk of suicide attempts by depressed patients, it may also be necessary to hospitalize the depressed patient with panic disorder when suicidal ideation is of clinical concern. The treatment of panic disorder along with the treatment of depression is then initiated on an inpatient basis. Similarly, patients with panic disorder frequently have comorbid substance use disorders, which can occasionally require inpatient detoxification. Once again, the treatment of panic can be initiated in the hospital before discharge to outpatient care. Rarely, hospitalization is required in very severe cases of panic disorder with agoraphobia when administration of outpatient treatment has been ineffective or is impractical. For example, a housebound patient may require more intensive and closely supervised CBT in the initial phase of therapy than that provided by outpatient care (178, 179).

B. FORMULATION OF A TREATMENT PLAN

Before treatment for panic disorder is initiated, a general medical and psychiatric evaluation should be conducted (15). Psychiatrists should consider potential general medical and substance-induced causes of panic symptoms, especially when caring for patients who have a new onset of symptoms. Diagnostic studies and laboratory tests should be guided by the psychiatrist's evaluation of the patient's condition and by the choice of treatment. Attention should be given to the patient's psychosocial stressors, social supports, and general living situation.

1. Psychiatric management

Once the diagnosis of panic disorder is made, the patient is informed of the diagnosis and educated about panic disorder, its clinical course, and its complications. Regardless of the ultimate treatment modality selected, it is important to reassure the patient that panic attacks reflect real physiologic events (e.g., the heart rate does increase, blood pressure usually goes up, and other physical changes occur) but that these changes are not dangerous acutely. To evaluate the frequency and nature of a patient's panic attacks, patients may be encouraged to monitor their symptoms by using techniques such as keeping a daily diary.

It is also extremely important when formulating the treatment plan to address the presence of any of the many conditions that are frequently comorbid with panic disorder. Continuing medical evaluation and management are a crucial part of the treatment plan. In some cases, treatment of these comorbid conditions may even take precedence over treatment of the panic attacks. For example, patients with serious substance abuse may need detoxification and substance abuse treatment before it is possible to institute treatment for panic disorder.

Regardless of the treatment modality, it is often helpful to involve family members and significant others when appropriate and possible. In many cases, panic disorder is not well understood by family members, who may accuse the patient of overreacting or even of malingering. In other cases, supportive and understanding family members may wish to participate in treatment by, for example, helping with exposure exercises. Educating family members and enlisting their help and support can be very helpful.

Family and supportive therapy may also be employed along with other psychosocial and pharmacologic treatments for panic disorder. This provides the necessary environment for improvement and helps resolve interpersonal issues that may have arisen as a direct result of panic attacks and avoidance behaviors.

Because patients with panic disorder often fear separations and being alone, many experience great comfort from having easy access to the treating psychiatrist. It is often important for a psychiatrist who treats patients with panic disorder to be very available to patients in the early phase of treatment, before the panic resolves. In general, these patients are very reassured by knowing their physicians are available. If the patient becomes overly dependent on the psychiatrist, the dependency should be addressed directly and nonjudgmentally in the treatment, rather than through physician unavailability. The psychiatrist should attend to the treatment of personality disorders in patients with panic disorder. Sometimes the symptoms of comorbid personality disorders are so prominent that they interfere with symptom-based treatment of panic disorder. In this case, psychodynamic psychotherapy may be indicated.

2. Choice of specific treatment modalities

As noted earlier, there are two methods that have been extensively studied and proven to be effective treatments for panic disorder: CBT and antipanic medication. Considerations that may help guide the choice between CBT and medication as the treatment modality include their comparable efficacies, differences in risks and benefits, differences in costs, the availability of clinicians trained in CBT, and patient preferences. The psychiatrist should remember that the best-studied treatments for panic disorder target specific symptoms, whereas the physician must treat the patient. This means that in some cases, less well-studied psychosocial treatment (e.g., psychodynamic psychotherapy, family therapy) may be the treatment of choice, for example, when symptoms of a personality disorder or extensive psychological conflicts are prominent in the clinical picture.

a. Considerations in choice of modality

1) Efficacy. Direct comparisons of the efficacy of CBT and antipanic medications have been conducted, and some CBT researchers have found CBT to be superior (30, 39), while some pharmacotherapy studies have shown medication to be superior (32). Results from a large four-site study documented that the two treatments perform equally well (180). This is in line with the conclusions of the NIMH consensus development panel in 1991 that either of these treatments could be considered standard and that there was not sufficient evidence that either was superior to the other (181).

2) Risks and benefits. The specific advantages and risks associated with CBT and pharmacotherapy may help guide the choice of which treatment to initiate. CBT lacks the adverse side effects of medications and the danger of developing physiological dependency on certain drugs. However, CBT requires patients to perform "homework" or confront feared situations, which approximately 10%–30% of patients have been found to be unwilling or unable to complete (19, 29, 30, 33). In addition, CBT may not be readily available to patients in some areas.

The advantages of pharmacotherapies include their ready availability, the need for less effort by the patient, and their more rapid onset (especially for benzodiazepines). Medications may be associated with a lower likelihood of psychological dependence on the therapist. Each class of antipanic medications (TCAs, MAOIs, SSRIs, and benzodiazepines) is associated with specific side effects, which must be considered (see discussion of choosing among the medication classes in section IV.B.2.b.2).

3) Costs. Several factors influence the costs of treatment. In the case of CBT, these factors include the duration and frequency of treatment, the ability to maintain treatment gains, and any requirements for additional psychosocial or pharmacologic treatment. For antipanic medications, factors affecting cost include the choice and dose of antipanic agent, the availability of generic preparations, duration of treatment, the probability of relapse following discontinuation, requirements for additional pharmacotherapy or psychosocial treatment, and costs of treating medication-related side effects.

4) Patient preferences. In most cases, the decision to use medication, CBT, another form of psychotherapy, or a combination of treatments is highly individualized. Informed patients may consider the evidence for a treatment's efficacy, particular advantages, risks and side effects, or costs.

b. Types of modalities

1) CBT and other psychotherapies. Specific elements of CBT are reviewed in section III.C.1.a. Panic-focused CBT is generally administered in weekly sessions for approximately 12 weeks. The patient must be willing to fulfill "homework" assignments that include breathing exercises, recording anxious cognitions, and confronting phobic situations.

Clinicians have often reported that sessions with significant others help to relieve stress on families caused by panic attacks and phobias in the patient and thereby promote a supportive environment for the patient, which may facilitate compliance with CBT and other treatments. Cognitive behavioral approaches have been conducted in group formats with results similar to those for individual treatment.

There is evidence that many patients with panic disorder have complicating comorbid axis I and/or axis II conditions. Psychodynamic psychotherapy may be useful in reducing symptoms or maladaptive behaviors in these associated conditions. Such a treatment may also be a helpful adjunct for patients with panic disorder treated with medication who continue to experience difficulty with psychosocial stressors.

Using other psychosocial treatments in conjunction with psychiatric management may be helpful in addressing certain comorbid disorders or environmental or psychosocial stressors. However, there have been no controlled studies to support the efficacy of psychosocial treatments other than CBT, when used alone, for the treatment of panic disorder. Therefore, supplementation with or replacement by either CBT or antipanic medications should be strongly considered if no significant improvement in the panic symptoms occurs within 6–8 weeks.

2) Medications. When pharmacotherapy has been selected, the choice of which class of medication to use may be informed by consideration of the relative efficacies of the various medication classes, differences in risks and benefits, differences in costs, and patient preferences, including the wish to conceive a child or continue with a pregnancy or nursing experience.

Because medications from all four classes—SSRIs, TCAs, benzodiazepines, and MAOIs—are roughly comparable in efficacy, the decision about which medication to choose for panic disorder mainly involves considerations of adverse side effects and cost. SSRIs are likely to be the best choice of pharmacotherapy for many patients with panic disorder because they lack significant cardiovascular and anticholinergic side effects and have no liability for physical dependency and subsequent withdrawal reactions.

The SSRIs carry a risk of sexual side effects and are also more expensive than tricyclics and benzodiazepines because generic preparations are not yet available. If cost is a consideration, it is important to note that tricyclics (particularly imipramine and clomipramine, for which most research has been conducted) and high-potency benzodiazepines (including alprazolam and clonazepam) are effective for panic disorder and that most patients can tolerate them. With tricyclics, consideration must be given to the possibility of cardiovascular and anticholinergic side effects. These are particularly troublesome for older patients and for patients with other medical problems. With benzodiazepines, consideration must be given to the fact that all of them will produce physical dependency in most patients. This may make it difficult for the patient to discontinue treatment. Also, benzodiazepines are generally contra-indicated for patients with current or past substance use disorders.

Because many patients with panic disorder are hypersensitive to antidepressant medications at treatment initiation, it is recommended that doses approximately half of those given to depressed patients at the beginning of treatment be used for patients with panic disorder initially. The dose is then increased to a full therapeutic dose over subsequent days and as tolerated by the patient. TCAs, SSRIs, and MAOIs generally take 4 to 6 weeks to become effective for panic disorder. For this reason, high-potency benzodiazepines may be useful in situations where very rapid control of symptoms is critical. Because of their side effects and the need for dietary restrictions, MAOIs are generally reserved for patients who do not respond to other treatments.

3) Combined medication and psychosocial treatment. The data regarding the efficacy of the combination of medications and CBT versus that of either modality alone are conflicting (66). Currently, it is not possible to identify which patients will benefit more from such combination therapy. Combining medication and CBT can be especially useful for patients with severe agoraphobia and for those who show an incomplete response to either treatment alone. In one study, combining psychodynamic psychotherapy with medication improved the long-term outcome of medication-treated patients (63). Psychodynamic psychotherapy is commonly used in conjunction with medication on the basis of a clinical consensus that it is effective for some patients.

3. Determining length of treatment

The acute phase of treatment with either CBT or medication generally lasts about 12 weeks. At the end of a successful acute phase, the patient should have markedly fewer and less intense panic attacks than before treatment. Ideally, panic attacks should be eliminated entirely. In addition, the patient should worry less about panic attacks and should experience minimal or no phobic avoidance. This is roughly the time required to realize the full benefit of either treatment.

After the acute phase of treatment with CBT, the frequency of visits is generally decreased, and they are eventually discontinued within several months. Some, but not all, studies indicate that long-term remission is possible, lasting several years after the completion of successful CBT. The efficacy of a second round of CBT for patients who relapse or "booster" CBT sessions for preventing relapse has not been studied.

There are very few systematic studies that indicate the optimal length of antipanic medication therapy. There is evidence that response to antipanic medication continues while the patient continues to take medication. Studies vary in the rate of relapse following medication discontinuation, but most show that relapse is common. It is generally believed, although not yet documented with research findings, that reinstitution of medication aborts relapse. The general recommendation has been to maintain medication treatment for at least 1 year after response and then to attempt discontinuation, with close follow-up of the patient from this point. Relapsing patients should then begin taking medication again. There is preliminary evidence that longer periods of initial treatment with medication may decrease the risk of relapse when the medication is stopped. It is not known whether continuing treatment with medication indefinitely for patients who relapse after discontinuation is beneficial.

Patients are likely to show some improvement with either medication or CBT within 6–8 weeks (although full response may take longer). Patients who show no improvement within 6–8 weeks with a particular treatment should be reevaluated with regard to diagnosis, the need for a different treatment, or the need for combined treatment. Patients who do not respond as expected to medication or CBT, or who have repeated relapses, should be evaluated for possible addition of a psychodynamic or other psychosocial intervention.

4. Use of benzodiazepines for early symptom control, in combination with a different treatment modality

Nonbenzodiazepine antipanic medication and CBT often take weeks before beneficial effects are realized, and some patients express an urgent need for a diminution of high levels of anticipatory anxiety and for some reduction in the severity of panic attacks. This can usually be accomplished by administering a benzodiazepine.

However, the potential benefits of benzodiazepines during the initial stages of treatment with another modality should be balanced against the potential risks. First, the patient may attribute all of the response he or she obtains in the course of treatment for panic disorder to the initial administration of the benzodiazepine. Even when antipanic medication or CBT has probably started to work, the patient may still believe that the benzodiazepine is the effective agent. The patient may then have difficulty discontinuing the benzodiazepine. Second, cognitive behavioral therapists and other clinicians are concerned that benzodiazepines may relieve anxiety to such an extent that the patient loses motivation to follow all of the steps of CBT. Finally, even after relatively brief periods of benzodiazepine treatment—often only a few weeks—some patients experience withdrawal reactions upon discontinuation. Such patients may believe that they are experiencing a relapse into panic disorder and have great difficulty stopping use of the benzodiazepine.

For these reasons, when benzodiazepines are used during the initial stages of treatment with another modality, patients should be reassured that more definitive treatment will be likely to work in a few weeks. Avoiding unnecessarily high doses of benzodiazepines and asking the patient to take these medications only when needed may help avoid the development of steady-state benzodiazepine levels and the risk of dependency.

V. Clinical Features Influencing Treatment

The following sections review data pertinent to the treatment of individuals with panic disorder who have specific clinical features that may alter the general treatment considerations that are discussed in section IV. These sections are necessarily brief and are not intended to stand alone as a set of treatment recommendations. The recommendations reviewed in section IV, including the use of psychiatric management, generally apply unless otherwise indicated.

A. PSYCHIATRIC FACTORS

1. Suicidality

Both older follow-up studies of anxiety disorders and more recent investigations of panic disorder have demonstrated a higher than average rate of suicide attempts in patients with a lifetime history of these disorders (9, 182, 183). In a large epidemiological study of over 18,000 adults, Weissman et al. (9) found that 20% of individuals with a history of panic disorder and 12% of those with a history of panic attacks had attempted suicide. A high risk of suicidal ideation and attempts in patients with panic disorder has been confirmed in several studies (184–186) but not in others examining uncomplicated panic disorder or controlling for comorbid conditions (187, 188). In addition, Fawcett et al. (189), in a study of 954 patients with major depression, found that the presence of comorbid panic attacks was one determinant of suicide in the first year of follow-up.

It remains unclear whether uncomplicated panic disorder, especially panic without agoraphobia, is associated with a high risk of suicide attempts (186–188, 190) and whether suicide attempts by individuals with panic disorder are actually related to or caused by panic symptoms, as opposed to being a result of comorbid conditions. Comorbid psychiatric disorders clearly increase the risk of suicide in patients with panic disorder. In particular, comorbid lifetime major depression, alcohol or substance abuse or dependence, personality disorders, and brief depressive symptoms increase the risk of suicide attempts, as do younger age, earlier onset of illness, greater severity of illness, and a past history of suicide attempts or psychiatric hospitalization (9, 183–185, 191, 192).

The high rate of suicide attempts by patients with panic disorder is of considerable clinical significance, even if most or all of the increased risk is attributable to lifetime comorbidity. The vast majority of patients with panic disorder have current or past comorbid axis I or axis II disorders. Thus, uncomplicated panic disorder is relatively uncommon. Furthermore, comorbid conditions may go undetected in busy clinical settings. Thus, it is important to be aware that patients presenting with panic disorder are at high risk for lifetime suicidal ideation and attempts. All patients presenting with panic attacks should be asked about suicidal ideation and past suicide attempts and about conditions likely to increase risk and to require specific treatment, such as depression and substance abuse. When significant depression and/or suicidal ideation exist, appropriate antidepressant therapy should be initiated and a decision made about whether the patient can be safely treated as an outpatient. When substance abuse is present, this must become a primary focus of clinical attention, and every effort to treat the substance abuse must be made.

2. Comorbid substance use disorder

In clinical and epidemiological studies, patients with panic disorder with or without agoraphobia have higher than average rates of cocaine, alcohol, and sedative abuse and dependence (193–196). Cocaine, other stimulants, and marijuana have been reported to precipitate panic attacks in adolescents and adults (197–199). Some individuals may self-medicate panic and anxiety symptoms by using alcohol and sedatives. However, heavy alcohol use, acute alcohol withdrawal, and more prolonged subacute withdrawal may cause or exacerbate panic (193, 200). Individuals who are ataxic and tremulous may not venture out because of their embarrassment, insecurity, or disability. These actions may mimic panic disorder or agoraphobia. Patients with both panic disorder and substance abuse or dependence have a poorer prognosis than those with either disorder alone (193, 200).

Since a significant proportion of patients presenting with panic attacks or agoraphobia have a history of substance abuse or dependence, which may cause or aggravate their symptoms, clinicians should be careful to screen for substance use disorders in this population. Flashbacks induced by current or past use of inhalants or hallucinogens can cause panic-disorder-type symptoms. Treatment of the substance use disorder is essential. It is unclear whether specific antipanic treatment is necessary for patients with primary substance abuse. Several panic attacks during the early weeks of abstinence, decreasing in frequency, often warrant no treatment other than support and reassurance until the attacks abate (201, 202). However, if the panic attacks continue and increase over several weeks, the diagnosis of panic disorder is warranted. If a patient is not relieved of ongoing panic attacks, it is likely that he or she will resume substance abuse (203–207). In treating panic symptoms in dually diagnosed patients, benzodiazepines should be avoided whenever possible, in favor of psychotherapy and/or antidepressants. A history of abuse of other substances, both licit and illicit, is associated with a higher prevalence of benzodiazepine abuse, a greater euphoric response to benzodiazepines, and a higher rate of unauthorized use of alprazolam during treatment for panic disorder (208, 209). The potential benefits of other medications for panic should be weighed against possible interactions with alcohol and other medications, resulting in, for instance, lowering of the seizure threshold (for tricyclics) or hyper- or hypotensive reactions (for MAOIs).

The use of a number of legal substances, such as nicotine, caffeine, and sympathomimetics (e.g., nasal decongestants), may also worsen panic attacks and interfere with treatment response (210–212).

3. Comorbid mood disorder

Panic disorder often coexists with bipolar disorder or unipolar depression. Bowen et al. (213) reported that of 108 patients with panic disorder, 11% had comorbid unipolar depression and 23% had comorbid bipolar disorder. Savino et al. (214) found that of 140 patients with panic, 23% had comorbid unipolar depression and 11% had comorbid bipolar disorder.

Many studies indicate that patients with panic disorder and comorbid mood disorders exhibit greater impairment, more hospitalizations, a higher rate of suicide attempts, and generally more psychopathology than patients with pure panic disorder (213). In addition, patients with panic disorder and comorbid affective disorders generally respond less well to traditional treatments for panic disorder.

A significant proportion of patients with panic disorder complain of overstimulation when treated with antidepressants (both tricyclics and SSRIs), and the attrition rate due to side effects or nonresponse is high. Such medications, therefore, are most efficaciously introduced at low doses and slowly increased. If both panic disorder and depression are present, it is important that a patient's treatment regimen include specific antipanic treatments.

4. Other anxiety disorders

Panic attacks are part of the hallmark cluster of symptoms in panic disorder, but they do occur in other illnesses. Patients with posttraumatic stress disorder (PTSD), obsessive-compulsive disorder (OCD), generalized anxiety disorder, and specific and social phobias also sometimes report occasional panic attacks. Identification of triggers for panic attacks is important, since a patient can be misdiagnosed with panic disorder and considered treatment resistant if this is not done.

Other comorbid anxiety disorders complicate the picture as well. PTSD, as just mentioned, may present with a series of panic attacks (215, 216), and PTSD patients may meet specific criteria for panic disorder concomitantly. In addition, patients with PTSD often present with PTSD, panic disorder, and a third or fourth disorder (217–223). More specific treatments may be required to offset other profound symptoms in PTSD. OCD is yet another anxiety disorder that may present concomitantly with panic disorder (224) and is frequently a diagnostic oversight, in part because of the reticence of patients to talk about their experiences. Because phobias and avoidant behavior are common in panic disorder, phobic disorders and panic disorder also frequently occur as comorbid conditions. They have similar responses to MAOIs, SSRIs, and perhaps other antidepressants. Specific phobias are more responsive to specific cognitive behavioral treatments than is the phobic avoidance associated with panic disorder. In summary, panic attacks may be experienced in several anxiety disorders, either as a response to specific triggers or as part of a complicated pattern of comorbid conditions that would require very specific, tailored multimodal therapy for optimal recovery. Although the pharmacotherapeutic considerations may be similar in these conditions, specificity of treatment may make the difference between full response, partial response, and perceived refractoriness.

5. Comorbid personality disorders

About 40% to 50% of patients with the diagnosis of panic disorder additionally meet the criteria for one or more axis II disorders (225–227).

The personality disorders most frequently observed in panic disorder patients are three from the anxious cluster: avoidant, obsessive-compulsive, and dependent (228–230). In addition, patients with panic disorder often show traits from other personality disorders, such as affective instability (from borderline personality disorder) and hypersensitivity to people (from paranoid personality disorder) (225).

Some studies suggest that patients with panic disorder and comorbid personality disorders may improve less or be subject to greater relapse following medication treatment (225, 228–231) or exposure therapy (42, 232–234). However, in one study (235), patients with panic disorder and comorbid personality disorders benefited as much from CBT as did patients with panic disorder without comorbid personality disorders, and in another study (236), there were no differences in treatment effect between patients with and without comorbid personality disorders after statistical adjustment for agoraphobic avoidance and frequency of panic attacks.

The therapist may need to spend more time with patients who have personality disorders in order to strengthen the therapeutic relationship and to develop a hierarchy of specific treatment goals. Psychodynamically informed management and/or formal psychodynamic treatment may be helpful for patients with panic disorder and personality disorders who have not responded to panic-focused treatments alone.

B. CONCURRENT GENERAL MEDICAL CONDITIONS

Panic attacks are associated with prominent physical symptoms and may be misinterpreted as general medical conditions by patients and/or physicians. Some general medical conditions (and/or effects of medications prescribed to treat them) may manifest themselves as panic symptoms, and general medical illness may be associated with comorbid panic disorder. A complete assessment for patients with panic disorder includes a general medical evaluation as delineated in the *Practice Guideline for Psychiatric Evaluation of Adults* (15). Such careful assessment, when results are negative, is reassuring for patients who fear serious physical illness. In the case of a patient who is diagnosed with a general medical condition, a decision must be made regarding the relationship between that condition and the panic disorder. If the medical condition or treatment is considered to be involved in the etiology of the panic symptoms, the treatment of panic disorder should be delayed until the general medical condition is treated and/or the medication discontinued. However, there may be a general medical condition that is not directly causing the panic disorder. Studies show that panic and other anxiety disorders are more prevalent in medically ill patients than in the population at large. Conditions that have been specifically associated with panic disorder, but not etiologically, include irritable bowel syndrome, migraine, and pulmonary disease (237–239). Acute onset of a wide range of medical conditions may also be associated with the development of an anxiety disorder. When a coexisting general medical condition is present, it is important to treat the panic disorder, since panic symptoms may exacerbate the associated general medical condition. Data from some studies suggest that panic disorder and phobic anxiety may increase the risk of mortality in patients with cardiovascular disease (182, 240). In general, treatment of panic disorder in patients with irritable bowel syndrome, pulmonary disease, or migraine is not different from treatment of uncomplicated panic disorder. In fact, studies have documented improvement in respiratory symptoms and amelioration of irritable bowel symptoms upon treatment with SSRIs, even when full-blown panic disorder is not present. If renal or liver damage is present or if there is general debilitation from general medical illness, the medication dose should be adjusted appropriately.

C. DEMOGRAPHIC VARIABLES

1. Child and adolescent population

The following section contains a brief overview of the available data regarding the treatment of children and adolescents with panic disorder. Unless stated otherwise, the general considerations discussed in section IV of this guideline apply to children; this is especially true of the importance of psychiatric management. Information and recommendations regarding the etiology, diagnosis, and assessment of panic disorder are beyond the scope of this section. The reader is referred to the American Academy of Child and Adolescent Psychiatry's *Practice Parameters for the Assessment and Treatment of Children and Adolescents With Anxiety Disorders* (241) for a more detailed discussion. Finally, the treatments reviewed are those for which the results of formal clinical trials have been published. Given the paucity of such data in the child and adolescent literature, many treatment plans will necessarily include components that are not well studied. For example, child and adolescent psychiatrists frequently find that a treatment plan requires attention to developmental issues (from psychological and physiological perspectives) and the involvement of multiple systems (e.g., schools, family, and community).

Panic disorder occurs in children and, more commonly, adolescents; panic disorder often is preceded by or co-occurs with separation anxiety disorder. This section reviews the literature on the treatment of pediatric panic disorder.

The literature on panic disorder in youth is considerably less robust than that for adults (242), and much controversy attends the relationship between separation anxiety disorder and panic disorder (243–245). Experts generally agree that treatment of panic disorder in children is similar to treatment of panic disorder in adults: cognitive behavioral psychotherapy and, where necessary, pharmacotherapy. Because family involvement in symptoms is common, family-based treatment strategies are often necessary. The literature regarding the psychodynamic treatment of children and adolescents tends to be focused on broader categories of anxiety disorders.

In one study of adolescents (246), panic disorder was reported to have a prevalence of 0.6% (girls, 0.7%; boys, 0.4%). Fewer than half of the young persons with panic disorder in this study had received treatment for panic disorder symptoms. The incidence of so-called limited-symptom panic attacks in young adolescents is somewhat greater and shows a steep increase with the onset of puberty (247). Panic disorder also occurs before puberty, although the true prevalence is unknown. Whether prepubertal or postpubertal, the presentation of panic disorder in young persons appears to be quite similar to that in adults, with the caveat that younger children show more separation anxiety symptoms (6).

Panic disorder is commonly accompanied by a variety of specific phobias, including fear of the dark, monsters, kidnappers, bugs, small animals, heights, and open or closed-in spaces. Nighttime fears, resistance to going to bed, difficulty falling asleep alone or sleeping through the night alone, and nightmares involving separation themes are not uncommon. These specific phobic symptoms may be common triggers for panic or separation anxiety and therefore are responsible for many of the avoidance and ritualized anxiety-reducing behaviors seen in patients with both separation anxiety disorder and panic disorder (242). Children with panic disorder also show high rates of comorbidity with other anxiety disorders and with depression (248). In younger children, separation anxiety disorder precedes depression in approximately two-thirds of the cases and may form the nidus for recurrent affective illness and panic disorder if left untreated (249).

The terms "school phobia" and "school refusal" are sometimes treated as reflecting panic disorder, even though not all children with school refusal show panic disorder and not all children with panic disorder manifest school refusal (250, 251). Moreover, while many school-refusing children do show significant separation anxiety, others are "phobic" school refusers, i.e., they are phobic of something within the school context and not fearful of leaving home or family (252, 253). Children also may refuse to go to school because of depressive disorders, conduct disorder, family problems, learning disabilities, or unrecognized mild retardation.

There is limited empirical research supporting the efficacy of any type of treatment of panic disorder in the pediatric population (242). Unfortunately, the pediatric literature primarily comprises uncontrolled studies, which are reviewed here.

Only a few published studies have addressed the treatment of panic disorder in children with cognitive behavioral techniques, and of these, there are no studies of contrasting groups. Only one study used a single-case design. Ollendick (254) applied standard treatments for panic disorder in adults (36, 255) to four adolescents with DSM-III-R panic disorder using a multiple-baseline-across-subjects design. In all cases, the panic attacks were eliminated, agoraphobia was reduced, and the ability to handle future "panico-genic" situations was enhanced.

Medication management strategies that are effective for adults with panic disorder have received anecdotal support for use with children and adolescents, but no treatment has shown conclusive support. Scattered case reports (256, 257) and case series (258, 259) suggest that standard TCAs, SSRIs, and the high-potency benzodiazepines alprazolam and clonazepam may be useful in treating pediatric panic disorder.

2. Geriatric population

Although anxiety symptoms and disorders are among the most common psychiatric ailments experienced by older adults, epidemiologic studies suggest that the prevalence of panic disorder in later life may be lower than that for midlife (260). A vigorous search for alternative and comorbid diagnoses, especially general medical conditions and effects of general medical pharmacologic agents, should be undertaken for elderly patients presenting with new panic symptoms. There have been few prospective clinical trials of anxiety disorder treatments for the elderly to document systematically the efficacy of standard medications and/or psychosocial treatments for this age group. If medication is used, the required dose may be lower than that for younger patients. The medication dose should be very low to begin, and medication increases should be slower and more limited than with younger adults. (Additional information will be provided in the forthcoming practice guideline on geriatric psychiatry.)

3. Gender

Panic disorder is more common in women for reasons that are not yet fully understood. In the Epidemiologic Catchment Area Study, the lifetime prevalence of panic disorder was twice as high in women as in men (261). The treatment of pregnant and nursing women raises certain specific concerns regarding the use of antipanic medications. A careful evaluation of the risks associated with frequently used medications has recently been reviewed by Altshuler et al. (262).

4. Cultural issues

Relatively little research has been done on anxiety disorders in African Americans. The National Institute of Mental Health Epidemiologic Catchment Area Study (263) and the National Comorbidity Survey (264) provide somewhat conflicting data on the prevalence of anxiety disorders. The Epidemiologic Catchment Area Study indicated that African Americans have a higher lifetime prevalence of agoraphobia but not panic disorder, while the National Comorbidity Survey found no racial differences in the prevalence of any anxiety disorder (264–266). Although the prevalences may be similar, racial differences in help seeking and symptom presentation may result in underrecognition and misdiagnosis. In one study (267), researchers identified panic disorder in 25% of a group of minority psychiatric outpatients of whom none had received this diagnosis from their clinicians. There is some evidence of a different clinical presentation of panic disorder in African Americans; specifically, there are associations with isolated sleep paralysis (268) and hypertension (269, 270). Studies show that African American patients in primary care report more severe somatic symptoms and have a higher prevalence of panic disorder than whites (271) and that African Americans are more likely to seek help in medical than in mental health facilities (272, 273).

VI. RESEARCH DIRECTIONS

A substantial amount of research has been devoted to the description of the phenomenology and treatment of panic disorder in recent years. Because of this, treatment of panic disorder is generally quite successful. These guidelines reveal, however, a number of areas in which further research would be most desirable.

Although the diagnosis of panic disorder is fairly straightforward, it is increasingly clear that a large proportion of patients with panic disorder also suffer from other anxiety disorders, depression, substance use disorders, and personality disorders. We have relatively little information on the optimal ways of treating these combinations of conditions or the extent to which comorbidity affects prognosis and whether the observed high rates of comorbidity are due to chance or fundamental overlaps in psychopathology. Hence, a thorough understanding of the relationship between panic disorder and other psychiatric disorders is needed.

In addition, while the start of a successful treatment for a patient with panic disorder may include reassurance that panic attacks are not medically catastrophic events, there are emerging data indicating that patients with phobic anxiety may have higher long-term rates of cardiovascular morbidity and mortality. It is not yet clear whether this association applies to individuals with a true diagnosis of panic disorder and, if it does, whether treatment diminishes the risk. Clearly, research about the long-term health risks that may be associated with panic disorder is needed.

We have very little scientifically accumulated information about panic disorder in childhood. It has been argued that separation anxiety in childhood is a precursor for panic disorder, but this has not been systematically substantiated. The epidemiology of panic disorder in childhood has not been well studied, nor has the optimal therapeutic approach been established.

These guidelines review a number of effective interventions for panic disorder, including pharmacotherapy and psychotherapy. Treatments are highly successful when measured in terms of the rate of panic attack blockade. On the other hand, studies continue to show that blocking panic attacks is only part of the solution to panic disorder and that many patients continue to suffer from associated features of the illness, including anticipatory anxiety and phobic avoidance. Very few long-term studies have been conducted to inform clinicians about how long treatment should last before there can be a reasonable certainty that response can be sustained. It is not known, for example, whether there is a length of medication exposure after which the patient with panic disorder will have a low chance for relapse. Similarly, it is not clear whether "booster" sessions of CBT are useful.

Even in selecting the first treatment for a new patient with panic disorder, there is uncertainty. Rigorous studies have shown that both medications and CBT are better than control treatments for panic disorder and approximately equal to each other. We do not yet know whether some individuals respond better to either CBT or medications and, if so, how to identify them. Further, it is not yet known whether combinations of medication and CBT are more effective than either treatment alone. Within the pharmacotherapy options, many medications have been shown to be effective, but few studies have elucidated whether there are advantages of one class over another, how benzodiazepines should properly be used if combined with antidepressants, or the best options for patients with refractory cases. CBT generally involves a "package" of several techniques, but it is not certain whether all of them are necessary or even beneficial.

Psychodynamic therapies and psychoanalysis are widely used for patients with panic disorder. Research is clearly needed to document the rates of response of patients with panic disorder to psychodynamically based treatments. This kind of research is clearly possible and deserves attention. Furthermore, whether psychodynamic treatments combined with medication or CBT offer any advantage over any of these treatments alone needs to be explored.

Finally, the treatment of any medical illness has a greater likelihood of success if it addresses fundamental pathological processes. Preclinical science is rapidly providing important insights into the biology of fear, and these findings must be translated into the clinical arena. This promises to open the way to highly specific antipanic therapies that will be improvements even over the very successful treatments we already have.

VII. Individuals and Organizations That Submitted Comments

David A. Adler, M.D.
Dick Baldwin, M.D.
James Ballenger, M.D.
Richard Balon, M.D.
Patricia L. Baltazar, Ph.D.
David H. Barlow, M.D., Ph.D.
Monica A. Basco, Ph.D.
William Bebchuk, M.D.
J. Gayle Beck, Ph.D.
Bernard D. Beitman, M.D.
Carl C. Bell, M.D.
Dinesh Bhugra, M.D.
Charles H. Blackinton, M.D.
Jack Blaine, M.D.
Barton J. Blinder, M.D., Ph.D.
David Brook, M.D.
Oliver G. Cameron, M.D., Ph.D.
Carlyle Chan, M.D.
Norman A. Clemens, M.D.
Christopher C. Colenda, M.D., M.P.H.
Michelle G. Craske, Ph.D.
Dorynne Czechowicz, M.D.
Jonathan Davidson, M.D.
Dave M. Davis, M.D.
Ted Dinan, M.D., Ph.D.
Kim A. Eagle, M.D.
James M. Ellison, M.D., M.P.H.
Frederick Engstrom, M.D.
Ann Maxwell Eward, Ph.D.
Harvey H. Falit, M.D.
Edward D. Frohlich, M.D.
Glen Gabbard, M.D.
David T. George, M.D.
William Goldman, M.D.
Sheila Hafter Gray, M.D.
Michael K. Greenberg, M.D.
William M. Greenberg, M.D.
George T. Grossberg, M.D.
Daniel W. Hicks, M.D.
Mac Horton, M.D.
Richard Justman, M.D.
Nalani V. Juthani, M.D.
Gary Kaplan, M.D.
Robert A. Kimmich, M.D.
Donald F. Klein, M.D.
Lawrence Kline, M.D.

Ronald R. Koegler, M.D.
Barry J. Landau, M.D.
Susan Lazar, M.D.
Henrietta Leonard, M.D.
Robert Liberman, M.D.
Francis G. Lu, M.D.
Henry Mallard, M.D.
Barton J. Mann, M.D.
V. Manohar, M.D.
John C. Markowitz, M.D.
Isaac Marks, M.D.
Ronald L. Martin, M.D.
Matis Mavissakalian, M.D.
Joseph Mawhinney, M.D.
Michael Mayo-Smith, M.D.
Christopher J. McLaughlin, M.D.
Barbara Milrod, M.D.
Jerome Motto, M.D.
Marvin Nierenberg, M.D.
Philip T. Ninan, M.D.
Russell Noyes, M.D.
David Osser, M.D.
Mark H. Pollack, M.D.
C. Alec Pollard, Ph.D.
Charles W. Portney, M.D.
Elizabeth Rahdert, Ph.D.
Penny Randall, M.D.
Michelle Riba, M.D.
Vaughn Rickert, Psy.D.
Barbara Rosenfeld, M.D.
Peter Roy-Byrne, M.D.
Pedro Ruiz, M.D.
Carlotta Schuster, M.D.
John J. Schwab, M.D.
Warren Seides, M.D.
Susan Simmons-Alling, M.S., R.N., C.S.
William Sledge, M.D.
Herbert Smokler, M.D.
David Spiegel, M.D.
Roger F. Suchyta, M.D.
Eva Szigethy, M.D., Ph.D.
Gerald Tarlow, Ph.D.
William R. Tatomer, M.D.
David M. Tobolowsky, M.D.
Mauricio Tohen, M.D., Dr.P.H.
Samuel M. Turner, Ph.D.

Robert M. Ward, M.D.
Naimah Weinberg, M.D.
Myrna Weissman, Ph.D.
Joseph Westermeyer, M.D.,
   M.P.H., Ph.D.
R. Reid Wilson, Ph.D.

Thomas Wise, M.D.
Earl Witenberg, M.D.
Sherwyn Woods, M.D., Ph.D.
Jesse H. Wright, M.D.
Roberto Zarate, M.D.
Howard Zonana, M.D.

American Academy of Addiction Psychiatry
American Academy of Child and Adolescent Psychiatry
American Academy of Neurology
American Academy of Pediatrics
American Association of Suicidology
American College of Cardiology
American Geriatric Society
American Nurses Association
American Psychoanalytic Association
American Psychosomatic Society
American Society of Addiction Medicine
American Society of Clinical Pathologists
Association for Academic Psychiatry
Association for the Advancement of Behavior Therapy
Association of Gay and Lesbian Psychiatrists
Baltimore/Washington Society for Psychoanalysis
Group for the Advancement of Psychiatry
National Institute on Drug Abuse
Royal College of Psychiatrists
Society for Adolescent Medicine

VIII. References

The following coding system is used to indicate the nature of the supporting evidence in the summary recommendations and references:

[A] *Randomized clinical trial.* A study of an intervention in which subjects are prospectively followed over time; there are treatment and control groups; subjects are randomly assigned to the two groups; both the subjects and the investigators are blind to the assignments.

[B] *Clinical trial.* A prospective study in which an intervention is made and the results of that intervention are tracked longitudinally; study does not meet standards for a randomized clinical trial.

[C] *Cohort or longitudinal study.* A study in which subjects are prospectively followed over time without any specific intervention.

[D] *Case-control study.* A study in which a group of patients is identified in the present and information about them is pursued retrospectively or backward in time.

[E] *Review with secondary data analysis.* A structured analytic review of existing data, e.g., a meta-analysis or a decision analysis.

[F] *Review.* A qualitative review and discussion of previously published literature without a quantitative synthesis of the data.

[G] *Other.* Textbooks, expert opinion, case reports, and other reports not included above.

1. American Psychiatric Association: Diagnostic and Statistical Manual of Mental Disorders, 4th ed (DSM-IV). Washington, DC, APA, 1994 [G]
2. Ballenger JC, Pecknold J, Rickels K, Sellers EM: Medication discontinuation in panic disorders. J Clin Psychiatry 1993; 54(Oct suppl):15–21, discussion 22–24 [F]
3. Katschnig H, Amering M, Stolk JM, Ballenger JC: Predictors of quality of life in a long-term follow-up study of panic disorder patients after a clinical drug trial. Psychopharmacol Bull 1996; 32:149–155 [C]
4. Roy-Byrne PP, Cowley DS: Course and outcome in panic disorder: a review of recent follow-up studies. Anxiety 1995; 1:150–160 [F]
5. Weissman MM, Bland RC, Canino GJ, Faravelli C, Greenwald S, Hwu HG, Joyce PR, Karam EG, Lee CK, Lellouch J, Lepine JP, Newman SC, Oakley-Browne MA, Rubio-Stipec M, Wells JE, Wickramaratne PJ, Wittchen HA, Yeh EK: The cross-national epidemiology of panic disorder. Arch Gen Psychiatry 1997; 54:305–309 [E]

6. Moreau D, Weissman MM: Panic disorder in children and adolescents: a review. Am J Psychiatry 1992; 149:1306–1314 [F]

7. Lesser IM, Rubin RT, Rifkin RP, Swinson RP, Ballenger JC, Burrows GD, DuPont RL, Noyes R, Pecknold JC: Secondary depression in panic disorder and agoraphobia, II: dimensions of depression symptomatology and their response to treatment. J Affect Disord 1989; 16:49–58 [B]

8. Klerman G, Weissman MM, Ouellette R, Johnson J, Greenwald S: Panic attacks in the community: social morbidity and health care utilization. JAMA 1991; 265:742–746 [E]

9. Weissman MM, Klerman GL, Markowitz JS, Ouellette R: Suicidal ideation and attempts in panic disorder and attacks. N Engl J Med 1989; 321:1209–1214 [C]

10. Markowitz JS, Weissman MM, Ouellette R, Lish JD, Klerman GL: Quality of life in panic disorder. Arch Gen Psychiatry 1989; 46:984–992 [B]

11. Knowles JA, Weissman MM: Panic disorder and agoraphobia, in American Psychiatric Press Review of Psychiatry, vol 14. Edited by Oldham JM, Riba MB. Washington, DC, American Psychiatric Press, 1995, pp 383–404 [G]

12. Goldstein RB, Wickramarante PJ, Horwath E, Weissman MM: Familial aggregation and phenomenology of "early"-onset (at or before age 20 years) panic disorder. Arch Gen Psychiatry 1997; 54:271–278 [C]

13. Kendler KS, Neale MC, Kessler RC, Heath AC, Eaves LJ: A test of the equal-environment assumption in twin studies of psychiatric illness. Behav Genet 1993; 23:21–27 [D]

14. Kendler KS, Neale MC, Kessler RC, Heath AC, Eaves LJ: Panic disorder in women: a population-based twin study. Psychol Med 1993; 23:387–406 [D]

15. American Psychiatric Association: Practice Guideline for Psychiatric Evaluation of Adults. Am J Psychiatry 1995; 152(Nov suppl):63–80 [G]

16. Cross-National Collaborative Panic Study SPI: Drug treatment of panic disorder: comparative efficacy of alprazolam, imipramine, and placebo. Br J Psychiatry 1992; 160:191–202, discussion 202–205; correction 1993; 161:724 [A]

17. Barlow DH, Craske MG: Mastery of Your Anxiety and Panic II. Albany, NY, Graywind Publications, 1994 [G]

18. Lydiard RB, Morton WA, Emmanuel NP, Zealberg JJ, Laraia MT, Stuart GW, O'Neil PM, Ballenger JC: Preliminary report: placebo-controlled, double-blind study of the clinical and metabolic effects of desipramine in panic disorder. Psychopharmacol Bull 1993; 29:183–188 [A]

19. Barlow DH, Craske MG, Cerney JA, Klosko JS: Behavioral treatment of panic disorder. Behavior Therapy 1989; 20:261–282 [A]

20. Clark DM, Salkovskis PM, Hackmann A, Middleton H, Anastasiades P, Gelder M: A comparison of cognitive therapy, applied relaxation and imipramine in the treatment of panic disorder. Br J Psychiatry 1994; 164:759–769 [A]

21. Beck AT, Sokol L, Clark DA, Berchick R, Wright F: A crossover study of focused cognitive therapy for panic disorder. Am J Psychiatry 1992; 149:778–783 [A]

22. Lydiard RB, Lesser IM, Ballenger JC, Rubin RT, Laraia M, DuPont R: A fixed-dose study of alprazolam 2 mg, alprazolam 6 mg, and placebo in panic disorder. J Clin Psychopharmacol 1992; 12:96–103 [A]

23. Fiegenbaum W: Long-term efficacy of ungraded versus graded massed exposure in agoraphobics, in Panic and Phobias 2: Treatments and Variables Affecting Course and Outcome. Edited by Hand I, Wittchen H-U. Berlin, Springer-Verlag, 1988, pp 83–88 [G]

24. Barlow DH: Anxiety and Its Disorders: The Nature and Treatment of Anxiety and Panic. New York, Guilford Press, 1988 [G]

25. Chambless DL, Gillis MM: Cognitive therapy of anxiety disorders. J Consult Clin Psychol 1993; 61:248–260 [E]

26. Clum GA, Suris R: A meta-analysis of treatments for panic disorder. J Consult Clin Psychol 1993; 61:317–326 [E]

27. Hofmann SG, Lehman CL, Barlow DH: How specific are specific phobias? J Behav Ther Exp Psychiatry 1997; 28:233–240 [C]

28. Margraf J, Gobel M, Schneider S: Cognitive-Behavioral Treatments for Panic Disorder, vol 5. Amsterdam, Swets and Zeitlinger, 1990 [G]

29. Craske MG, Brown TA, Barlow DH: Behavioral treatment of panic disorder: a two-year follow-up. Behavior Therapy 1991; 22:289–304 [D]

30. Klosko JS, Barlow DH, Tassinari R, Cerny JA: A comparison of alprazolam and behavior therapy in treatment of panic disorder. J Consult Clin Psychol 1990; 58:77–84 [A]

31. Clark DB, Agras WS: The assessment and treatment of performance anxiety in musicians. Am J Psychiatry 1991; 148:598–605 [A]

32. Black DW, Wesner R, Bowers W, Gabel J: A comparison of fluvoxamine, cognitive therapy and placebo in the treatment of panic disorder. Arch Gen Psychiatry 1993; 50:44–50 [A]

33. Telch MJ, Lucas JA, Schmidt NB, Hanna HH, Jaimez LT, Lucas RA: Group cognitive-behavioral treatment of panic disorder. Behav Res Ther 1993; 31:279–287 [A]

34. Craske MG, Rodriguez BI: Behavioral treatment of panic disorders and agoraphobia. Prog Behav Modif 1994; 29:1–26 [A]

35. Shear MK, Pilkonis PA, Cloitre M, Leon AC: Cognitive behavioral treatment compared with nonprescriptive treatment of panic disorder. Arch Gen Psychiatry 1994; 51:395–401 [A]

36. Ost LG, Westling BE: Applied relaxation vs cognitive behavior therapy in the treatment of panic disorder. Behav Res Ther 1995; 33:145–158 [A]

37. Ost LG, Westling BE, Hellstrom K: Applied relaxation exposure in vivo and cognitive methods in the treatment of panic disorder with agoraphobia. Behav Res Ther 1993; 31:383–394 [A]

38. van den Hout M, Arntz A, Hoekstra R: Exposure reduced agoraphobia but not panic and cognitive therapy reduced pain but not agoraphobia. Behav Res Ther 1994; 32:447–451 [A]

39. Marks IM, Swinson RP, Basoglu M: Alprazolam and exposure alone and combined in panic disorder with agoraphobia. Br J Psychiatry 1993; 162:776–787 [B]

40. Swinson RP, Soulios C, Cox BJ, Kuch K: Brief treatment of emergency room patients with panic attacks. Am J Psychiatry 1992; 149:944–946 [A]

41. Swinson RP, Fergus KD, Cox BJ, Wickwire K: Efficacy of telephone-administered behavioral therapy for panic disorder. Behav Res Ther 1995; 33:465–469 [B]

42. Fava GA, Zielezny M, Savron G, Grandi S: Long-term effects of behavioural treatment for panic disorder with agoraphobia. Br J Psychiatry 1995; 166:87–92 [B]

43. Brown TA, Barlow DH: Long term outcome of cognitive behavioral treatment of panic disorder. J Consult Clin Psychol 1995; 63:754–765 [B]

44. O'Sullivan G, Marks IM: Long-term outcome of phobic and obsessive compulsive disorders after exposure: a review chapter, in The Treatment of Anxiety: Handbook of Anxiety, vol 4. Edited by Noyes R, Roth M, Burrows G. Amsterdam, Elsevier, 1990, pp 82–108 [G]

45. Barlow DH: Cognitive-behavioral therapy for panic disorder: current status. J Clin Psychiatry 1997; 58(suppl 2):32–36 [F]

46. Shear MK, Barlow D, Gorman J, Woods S: Multicenter treatment study of panic disorder. Presented at the 36th annual meeting of the American College of Neuropsychopharmacology, Kamuela, Hawaii, Dec 8–12, 1997 [A]

47. Neron S, Lacroix D, Chaput Y: Group vs individual cognitive behaviour therapy in panic disorder: an open clinical trial with a six month follow-up. Can J Behavioral Sci 1995; 27:379–392 [C]

48. Cerny JA, Barlow DH, Craske MG, Himadi WG: Couples treatment of agoraphobia: a two-year follow-up. Behavior Therapy 1987; 18:401–415 [C]

49. Craske MG, Rowe M, Lewin M, Noriega-Dimitri R: Interoceptive exposure versus breathing retraining within cognitive-behavioural therapy for panic disorder with agoraphobia. Br J Clin Psychol 1997; 36(part 1):85–99 [A]

50. Hoffart A, Thornes K, Hedley LM: DSM-III-R axis I and II disorders in agoraphobic inpatients before and after psychosocial treatment. Psychiatry Res 1995; 56:1–9 [C]

51. Lidren D, Watkins P, Gould R, Clum G, Asterino M, Tulloch H: A comparison of bibliotherapy and group therapy in the treatment of panic disorder. J Consult Clin Psychol 1994; 62:865–869 [B]

52. Carter MM, Turovsky J, Barlow DH: Interpersonal relationships in panic disorder with agoraphobia: a review of empirical evidence. Clin Psychol: Science and Practice 1994; 1:25–34 [F]

53. Spiegel DA, Bruce TJ, Gregg SF, Nuzzarello A: Does cognitive behavior therapy assist slow-taper alprazolam discontinuation in panic disorder? Am J Psychiatry 1994; 151: 876–881 [A]

54. Otto MW, Pollack MH, Sachs GS, Reiter SR, Meltzer-Brody S, Rosenbaum JF: Discontinuation of benzodiazepine treatment: efficacy of cognitive-behavioral therapy for patients with panic disorder. Am J Psychiatry 1993; 150:1485–1490 [A]

55. Spiegel DA, Bruce TJ: Benzodiazepines and exposure-based cognitive behavior therapies for panic disorder: conclusion from combined treatment trials. Am J Psychiatry 1997; 154:773–781 [F]

56. Milrod B, Busch F, Cooper A, Shapiro T: Manual of Panic-Focused Psychodynamic Psychotherapy. Washington, DC, American Psychiatric Press, 1997 [G]

57. Kohut H: Thoughts on narcissism and narcissistic rage. Psychoanal Study Child 1972; 27:360–400 [G]

58. Bash M: Doing Brief Psychotherapy. New York, Basic Books, 1995 [G]

59. Gray JA: The neuropsychiatry of anxiety. Br J Psychol 1978; 69:417–434 [G]

60. Sifneos PE: The current status of individual short-term dynamic psychotherapy and its future: an overview. Am J Psychother 1984; 38:472–483 [G]

61. Sifneos PE: Short-term dynamic psychotherapy for patients with physical symptomatology. Psychother Psychosom 1984; 42:48–51 [F]

62. Shear MK: Psychotherapeutic issues in long-term treatment of anxiety disorder patients. Psychiatr Clin North Am 1995; 18:885–894 [F]

63. Wiborg IM, Dahl AA: Does brief dynamic psychotherapy reduce the relapse rate of panic disorder? Arch Gen Psychiatry 1996; 53:689–694 [A]

64. Beitman BD, Goldfried MR, Norcross JC: The movement toward integrating the psychotherapies: an overview. Am J Psychiatry 1989; 146:138–147 [G]

65. Shear MK, Weiner K: Psychotherapy for panic disorder. J Clin Psychiatry 1997; 58(suppl 2):38–43 [G]

66. Zitrin CM, Klein DF, Woerner MG: Treatment of agoraphobia with group exposure in vivo and imipramine. Arch Gen Psychiatry 1980; 37:63–72 [A]

67. Zitrin CM, Klein DF, Woerner MG, Ross DC: Treatment of phobias, I: comparison of imipramine hydrochloride and placebo. Arch Gen Psychiatry 1983; 40:125–138 [A]

68. Marks IM, Gray S, Cohen D, Hill R, Mawson D, Ramm E, Stern RS: Imipramine and brief therapist-aided exposure in agoraphobics having self-exposure homework. Arch Gen Psychiatry 1983; 40:153–162 [A]

69. Mavissakalian M, Michelson L, Dealy RS: Pharmacological treatment of agoraphobia: imipramine vs imipramine with programmed practice. Br J Psychiatry 1983; 143:348–355 [A]

70. Telch MJ, Agras WS, Taylor CB, Roth WT, Gallen CC: Combined pharmacological and behavioral treatment for agoraphobia. Behav Res Ther 1985; 23:325–335 [A]

71. Mavissakalian M, Michelson L: Relative and combined effectiveness of therapist-assisted in vivo exposure and imipramine. J Clin Psychiatry 1986; 47:117–122 [B]

72. Mavissakalian M, Michelson L: Two-year follow-up of exposure and imipramine treatment of agoraphobia. Am J Psychiatry 1986; 143:1106–1112 [B]

73. Oehrberg S, Christiansen PE, Behnke K: Paroxetine in the treatment of panic disorder: a randomized double-blind placebo-controlled study. Br J Psychiatry 1995; 167:374–379 [A]

74. Pollack MH, Otto MW, Kaspi SP, Hammerness PG, Rosenbaum JF: Cognitive behavior therapy for treatment-refractory panic disorder. J Clin Psychiatry 1994; 55:200–205 [B]

75. Nagy LM, Krystal JH, Woods SW: Clinical and medication outcome after short-term alprazolam and behavioral group treatment of panic disorder: 2.5 year naturalistic follow-up. Arch Gen Psychiatry 1989; 46:993–999 [B, C]

76. Kabat-Zinn J, Massion AO, Kristeller J, Peterson LG, Fletcher KE, Pbert L, Lenderking WR, Santorelli SF: Effectiveness of a meditation-based stress reduction program in the treatment of anxiety disorders. Am J Psychiatry 1992; 149:936–943 [B]

77. Miller JJ, Fletcher K, Kabat-Zinn J: Three-year follow-up and clinical implications of a mindfulness meditation-based stress reduction intervention in the treatment of anxiety disorders. Gen Hosp Psychiatry 1995; 17:192–200 [D]

78. Buglass D, Clarke J, Henderson AS, Kreitman N: A study of agoraphobic housewives. Psychol Med 1977; 7:73–86 [D]

79. Arrindell WA, Emmelkamp PM: Marital adjustment, intimacy and needs in female agoraphobics and their partners: a controlled study. Br J Psychiatry 1986; 149:592–602; correction 1987; 150:273 [D]

80. Lange A, van Dyck R: The function of agoraphobia in the marital relationship. Acta Psychiatr Scand 1992; 85:89–93 [E]

81. Hafner RJ: Predicting the effects on husbands of behaviour therapy for wives' agoraphobia. Behav Res Ther 1984; 22:217–226 [C]

82. Milton F, Hafner J: The outcome of behavior therapy for agoraphobia in relation to marital adjustment. Arch Gen Psychiatry 1979; 36:807–811 [B]

83. Jacobson NS, Holtzworth-Monroe A, Schmaling KB: Marital therapy and spouse involvement in the treatment of depression, agoraphobia, and alcoholism. J Consult Clin Psychol 1989; 57:5–10 [F]

84. Himadi WG, Cerny JA, Barlow DH, Cohen S, O'Brien GT: The relationship of marital adjustment to agoraphobia treatment outcome. Behav Res Ther 1986; 24:107–115 [C]

85. Barlow DH, O'Brien GT, Last CG: Couples treatment of agoraphobia. Behavior Therapy 1984; 15:41–58 [C]

86. Arnow BA, Taylor CB, Agras WS: Enhancing agoraphobia treatment outcome by changing couple communication patterns. Behavior Therapy 1985; 16:452–467 [C]

87. Lydiard RB, Pollack MH, Judge R, Michelson D, Tamura R: Fluoxetine in panic disorder: a placebo-controlled study. Presented at the 10th Congress of the European College of Neuropsychopharmacology, Vienna, Sept 13–17, 1997 [A]

88. Gorman JM, Liebowitz MR, Fyer AJ, Goetz D, Campeas RB, Fyer MR, Davies SO, Klein DF: An open trial of fluoxetine in the treatment of panic disorder. J Clin Psychopharmacol 1987; 7:319–332 [B]

89. Schneier FR, Liebowitz MR, Davies SO, Fairbanks J, Hollander E, Campeas R, Klein DF: Fluoxetine in panic disorder. J Clin Psychopharmacol 1990; 10:119–121 [B]

90. Wolkow R, Apter J, Clayton A, Coryell W, Cunningham L, McEntee W, O'Hair D, Pollack M, Rausch J, Stewart R, Weisler R: Double-blind flexible dose study of sertraline and placebo in patients with panic disorder. Presented at the XX Congress of the Collegium Internationale Neuro-Psychopharmacologicum, Melbourne, Australia, June 23–27, 1996 [A]

91. Baumel B, Bielski R, Carman J, Hegel M, Houck C, Linden R, Nakra B, Ota K, Pohl R, Wolkow R: Double-blind comparison of sertraline and placebo in patients with panic disorder. Ibid [A]

92. Ballenger JC, Wheadon DE, Steiner M, Bushnell W, Gergel IP: Double-blind, fixed-dose, placebo-controlled study of paroxetine in the treatment of panic disorder. Am J Psychiatry 1998; 155:36–42 [A]

93. LeCrubier Y, Bakker A, Dunbar G, Judge R: A comparison of paroxetine, clomipramine and placebo in the treatment of panic disorder. Acta Psychiatr Scand 1997; 95:145–152 [A]

94. Hoehn-Saric R, McLeod DR, Hipsley PA: Effect of fluvoxamine on panic disorder. J Clin Psychopharmacol 1993; 13:321–326 [B]

95. de Beurs E, van Balkom AJ, Lange A, Koele P, van Dyck R: Treatment of panic disorder with agoraphobia: comparison of fluvoxamine, placebo, and psychological panic management combined with exposure and of exposure in vivo alone. Am J Psychiatry 1995; 152:683–691 [B]

96. Westenberg HG, den Boer JA: Selective monoamine uptake inhibitors and a serotonin antagonist in the treatment of panic disorder. Psychopharmacol Bull 1989; 25:119–123 [B]

97. Wade AG, Lepola U, Koponen HJ, Pedersen V, Pedersen T: The effect of citalopram in panic disorder. Br J Psychiatry 1997; 170:549–553 [A]

98. Boyer W: Serotonin uptake inhibitors are superior to imipramine and alprazolam in alleviating panic attacks: a meta-analysis. Int Clin Psychopharmacol 1995; 10:45–49 [E]

99. Lejoyeux M, Ades J: Antidepressant discontinuation: a review of the literature. J Clin Psychiatry 1997; 58(July suppl): 11–16 [G]

100. Louie AK, Lewis TB, Lannon RA: Use of low-dose fluoxetine in major depression and panic disorder. J Clin Psychiatry 1993; 54:435–438 [C]

101. Emmanuel NP, Crosby C, Ware MR, Lydiard RB: The efficacy of once-a-week fluoxetine dosing in the treatment of panic disorder, in 1996 Annual Meeting New Research Program and Abstracts. Washington, DC, American Psychiatric Association, 1996, p 252 [G]

102. DuBoff E, England D, Ferguson JM, Londborg PD, Rosenthal MH, Smith W, Weise C, Wolkow RM: Sertraline in the treatment of panic disorder. Presented at the 8th Congress of the European College of Neuropsychopharmacology, Venice, Sept 30 to Oct 4, 1995 [A]

103. Gergel I, Burnham D, Kumar R: Treatment of panic disorder with paroxetine. Presented at the 6th World Congress of Biological Psychiatry, Nice, France, June 22–27, 1997 [A]

104. Klein D: Delineation of two drug-responses for anxiety syndromes. Psychopharmacologia 1964; 5:397–408 [A]

105. Uhlenhuth EH, Matuzas W, Glass RM, Easton C: Response of panic disorder to fixed doses of alprazolam or imipramine. J Affect Disord 1989; 17:261–270 [A]

106. Modigh K, Westberg P, Eriksson E: Superiority of clomipramine over imipramine in the treatment of panic disorder: a placebo-controlled trial. J Clin Psychopharmacol 1992; 12:251–261 [A]

107. Andersch S, Rosenberg NK, Kullingsjo H, Ottoson JQ, Hanson L, Lorentzen K, Mellergard M, Rasmussen S, Rosenberg R: Efficacy and safety of alprazolam, imipramine, and placebo in treating panic disorder: a Scandinavian multicenter study. Acta Psychiatr Scand Suppl 1991; 365:18–27 [A]

108. Mavissakalian M, Perel J: Imipramine in the treatment of agoraphobia: dose-response relationships. Am J Psychiatry 1985; 142:1032–1036 [A]

109. Mavissakalian MR, Perel JM: Imipramine dose-response relationship in panic disorder with agoraphobia. Arch Gen Psychiatry 1989; 46:127–131 [A]

110. Mavissakalian MR, Perel JM: Imipramine treatment of panic disorder with agoraphobia: dose ranging and plasma level-response relationships. Am J Psychiatry 1995; 152:673–682 [A]

111. Maier W, Roth SM, Argyle N, Buller R, Lavori P, Brandon S, Benkert O: Avoidance behaviour: a predictor of the efficacy of pharmacotherapy in panic disorder? Eur Arch Psychiatry Clin Neurosci 1991; 241:151–158 [A]

112. Cassano GB, Toni C, Musetti L: Treatment of panic disorder, in Synaptic Transmission. Edited by Biggio G, Concas A, Costa E. New York, Raven Press, 1992, pp 449–461 [A]

113. Curtis GC, Massana J, Udina C, Ayuso JL, Cassano GB, Perugi G: Maintenance drug therapy of panic disorder. J Psychiatr Res 1993; 27(suppl 1):127–142 [A]

114. Keller MB, Lavori PW, Goldenberg IM, Baker LA, Pollack MH, Sachs GS, Rosenbaum JF, Deltito JA, Leon A, Shear K, Klerman GL: Influence of depression on the treatment of panic disorder with imipramine, alprazolam, imipramine. J Affect Disord 1993; 28:27–38 [A]

115. Woods S, Nagy LM, Koleszar AS, Krystal JH, Heninger GR, Charney DS: Controlled trial of alprazolam supplementation during imipramine treatment of panic disorder. J Clin Psychopharmacol 1991; 12:32–38 [A]

116. Mellergard M, Lorentzen K, Bech P, Ottoson JQ, Rosenberg R: A trend analysis of changes during treatment of panic disorder with alprazolam and imipramine. Acta Psychiatr Scand Suppl 1991; 365:28–32 [A]

117. Pollack MH, Otto MW, Sachs GS, Leon A, Shear MK, Deltito JA, Keller MB, Rosenbaum JF: Anxiety psychopathology predictive of outcome in patients with panic disorder and depression treated with imipramine, alprazolam, and placebo. J Affect Disord 1994; 30:273–281 [A]

118. Den Boer JA, Westenberg HG: Effect of a serotonin and noradrenaline uptake inhibitor in panic disorder: a double-blind comparative study with fluvoxamine and maprotiline. Int Clin Psychopharmacol 1988; 3:59–74 [B]

119. Cassano GB, Petracca A, Perugi G, Nisita C, Musetti L, Mengali F, McNair DM: Clomipramine for panic disorder, I: the first 10 weeks of a long-term comparison with imipramine. J Affect Disord 1988; 14:123–127 [B]

120. Monteiro WO, Noshirvani HF, Marks IM: Anorgasmia from clomipramine in obsessive-compulsive disorder: a controlled trial. Br J Psychiatry 1987; 151:107–112 [B]

121. Mavissakalian M, Perel JM: Clinical experiments in maintenance and discontinuation of imipramine therapy in panic disorder with agoraphobia. Arch Gen Psychiatry 1992; 49:318–323 [B]

122. Mavissakalian M, Perel JM: Protective effects of imipramine maintenance treatment in panic disorder with agoraphobia. Am J Psychiatry 1992; 149:1053–1057 [B]

123. Sheehan DV: Tricyclic antidepressants in the treatment of panic and anxiety disorders. Psychosomatics 1986; 27:10–16 [F]

124. Fyer AJ, Liebowitz MR, Gorman JM, Campeas R, Levin A, Davies SO, Goetz D, Klein DF: Discontinuation of alprazolam treatment in panic patients. Am J Psychiatry 1987; 144:303–308 [B]

125. Klerman GL: Overview of the Cross-National Collaborative Panic Study. Arch Gen Psychiatry 1988; 45:407–412 [F]

126. Dunner DL, Ishiki D, Avery DH, Wilson LG, Hyde TS: Effect of alprazolam and diazepam in anxiety and panic attacks in panic disorder: a controlled study. J Clin Psychiatry 1986; 47:458–460 [B]

127. Ballenger JC, Burrows GD, DuPont RL Jr, Lesser IM, Noyes R Jr, Pecknold JC, Rifkin A, Swinson RP: Alprazolam in panic disorder and agoraphobia: results from a multicenter trial, I: efficacy in short-term treatment. Arch Gen Psychiatry 1988; 45:413–422 [A]

128. Tesar GE, Rosenbaum JF, Pollack MH, Otto MW, Sachs GS, Herman JB, Cohen LS, Spier SA: Double-blind, placebo-controlled comparison of clonazepam and alprazolam for panic disorder. J Clin Psychiatry 1991; 52:69–76 [A]

129. Schweizer E, Rickels K, Weiss S, Zavodnick S: Maintenance drug treatment of panic disorder, I: results of a prospective, placebo-controlled comparison of alprazolam and imipramine. Arch Gen Psychiatry 1993; 50:51–60 [A]

130. Dager SR, Roy-Byrne P, Hendrickson H, Cowley DS, Avery DH, Hall KC, Dunner DL: Long-term outcome of panic states during double-blind treatment and after withdrawal of alprazolam and placebo. Ann Clin Psychiatry 1992; 4:251–258 [A]

131. Chouinard G, Annable L, Fontaine R, Solyom L: Alprazolam in the treatment of generalized anxiety and panic disorders: a double-blind placebo-controlled study. Psychopharmacology (Berl) 1982; 77:229–233 [B]

132. McNair DM, Kahn RJ: Imipramine compared with a benzodiazepine for agoraphobia, in Anxiety: New Research and Changing Concepts. Edited by Klein DF, Rabkin J. New York, Raven Press, 1981, pp 69–80 [B]

133. Noyes RJ, Anderson DJ, Clancy J, Crowe RR, Slymen DJ, Ghoneim MM, Hinrichs JV: Diazepam and propranolol in panic disorder and agoraphobia. Arch Gen Psychiatry 1984; 41:287–292 [A]

134. Schweizer E, Rickels K: Failure of buspirone to manage benzodiazepine withdrawal. Am J Psychiatry 1986; 143:1590–1592 [B]

135. Schweizer E, Case WG, Rickels K: Benzodiazepine dependence and withdrawal in elderly patients. Am J Psychiatry 1989; 146:529–531 [B]

136. Schweizer E, Clary C, Dever AI, Mandos LA: The use of low-dose intranasal midazolam to treat panic disorder: a pilot study. J Clin Psychiatry 1992; 53:19–22 [B]

137. Charney DS, Woods SW: Benzodiazepine treatment of panic disorder: a comparison of alprazolam and lorazepam. J Clin Psychiatry 1989; 50:418–423 [B]

138. Pyke RE, Greenberg HS: Double-blind comparison of alprazolam and adinazolam for panic and phobia disorders. J Clin Psychopharmacol 1989; 9:15–21 [B]

139. Savoldi F, Somenzini G, Ecari U: Etizolam versus placebo in the treatment of panic disorder with agoraphobia: a double-blind study. Curr Med Res Opin 1990; 12:185–190 [A]

140. Beaudry P, Fontaine R, Chouinard G: Bromazepam, another high-potency benzodiazepine for panic attacks (letter). Am J Psychiatry 1984; 141:464–465 [G]

141. Noyes R, Borrows GD, Reich JH, Judd FK, Garvey M, Morman TR, Cook BL, Marriot P: Diazepam versus alprazolam for the treatment of panic disorder. J Clin Psychiatry 1996; 57:349–355 [A]

142. Benzodiazepine Dependence, Toxicity, and Abuse: A Task Force Report of the American Psychiatric Association. Washington, DC, APA, 1990 [G]

143. Rickels K, Schweizer E, Weiss S, Zavodnick S: Maintenance drug treatment for panic disorder, II: short- and long-term outcome after drug taper. Arch Gen Psychiatry 1993; 50:61–68 [B]

144. Klein E, Colin V, Stolk J, Lenox RH: Alprazolam withdrawal in patients with panic disorder and generalized anxiety disorder: vulnerability and effect of carbamazapine. Am J Psychiatry 1994; 151:1760–1766 [A]

145. Noyes R Jr, Garvey MJ, Cook B, Suelzer M: Controlled discontinuation of benzodiazepine treatment for patients with panic disorder. Am J Psychiatry 1991; 148:517–523 [B]

146. Pecknold JC, Swinson RP: Taper withdrawal studies with alprazolam inpatients with panic disorder and agoraphobia. Psychopharmacol Bull 1986; 22:173–176 [A]

147. Rosenbaum JF, Moroz G, Bowden CL: Clonazepam in the treatment of panic disorder with or without agoraphobia: a dose-response study of efficacy, safety, and discontinuance. J Clin Psychopharmacol 1997; 17:390–400 [A]

148. Lesser IM, Lydiard RB, Antal E, Rubin RT, Ballenger JC, DuPont R: Alprazolam plasma concentrations and treatment response in panic disorder and agoraphobia. Am J Psychiatry 1992; 149:1556–1562 [A]

149. Greenblatt DJ, Harmatiz JS, Shader RI: Plasma alprazolam concentrations: relation to efficacy and side effects in the treatment of panic disorder. Arch Gen Psychiatry 1993; 50: 715–722 [B]

150. Lepola UM, Rimon RH, Riekkinen PJ: Three-year follow-up of patients with panic disorder after short-term treatment with alprazolam and imipramine. Int Clin Psychopharmacol 1993; 8:115–118 [B]

151. Sheehan DV, Claycomb JB, Kouretas N: Monoamine oxidase inhibitors: prescription and patient management. Int J Psychiatry Med 1980–1981; 10:99–121 [G]

152. American Psychiatric Association: Diagnostic and Statistical Manual of Mental Disorders, 2nd ed (DSM-II). Washington, DC, APA, 1968 [G]

153. Bakish D, Saxena BM, Bowen R, D'Souza J: Reversible monoamine oxidase-A inhibitors in panic disorder. Clin Neuropsychopharmacol 1993; 16(suppl 2):S77–S82 [A]

154. Garcia-Borreguero D, Lauer CJ, Ozdaglar A, Wiedemann K, Holsboer F, Krieg JC: Brofaromine in panic disorder: a pilot study with a new reversible inhibitor of monoamine oxidase-A. Pharmacopsychiatry 1992; 25:261–264 [B]

155. van Harten J: Clinical pharmacokinetics of selective serotonin reuptake inhibitors. Clin Pharmacokinet 1993; 24:203–220 [F]

156. Pollack MH, Worthington JJ, Otto MW, Maki KM, Smoller JW, Manfro GG, Rudolph R, Rosenbaum JF: Venlafaxine for panic disorder: results from a double-blind, placebo-controlled study. Psychopharmacol Bull 1996; 32:667–670 [A]

157. Geracioti JD: Venlafaxine treatment of panic disorder: a case series. J Clin Psychiatry 1995; 56:408–410 [G]

158. Charney DS, Woods SW, Goodman WK, Rifkin B, Kinch M, Aiken B, Quadrino LM, Heninger GR: Drug treatment of panic disorder: the comparative efficacy of imipramine, alprazolam, and trazodone. J Clin Psychiatry 1986; 47:580–586 [B]

159. Mavissakalian M, Perel J, Bowler K, Dealy R: Trazodone in the treatment of panic disorder and agoraphobia with panic attacks. Am J Psychiatry 1987; 144:785–787 [B]

160. Sheehan DV, Davidson J, Manschreck T, Van Wyck Fleet J: Lack of efficacy of a new antidepressant (bupropion) in the treatment of panic disorder with phobias. J Clin Psychopharmacol 1983; 3:28–31 [G]

161. Zajecka JM: The effect of nefazodone on comorbid anxiety symptoms associated with depression: experience in family practice and psychiatric outpatient settings. J Clin Psychiatry 1996; 57(2 suppl):10–14 [A]

162. DeMartinis NA, Schweizer E, Rickels K: An open-label trial of nefazodone in high comorbidity panic disorder. J Clin Psychiatry 1996; 57:245–248 [B]

163. Keck PE Jr, McElroy SL, Friedman LM: Valproate and carbamazepine in the treatment of panic and posttraumatic stress disorders, withdrawal states, and behavioral dyscontrol syndromes. J Clin Psychopharmacol 1992; 12(1 suppl):36S–41S [F]

164. Uhde TW, Stein MB, Post RM: Lack of efficacy of carbamazepine in the treatment of panic disorder. Am J Psychiatry 1988; 145:1104–1109 [B]

165. Lum M, Fontaine R, Elie R, Ontiveros A: Divalproex sodium's antipanic effect in panic disorder: a placebo-controlled study. Biol Psychiatry 1990; 27(9A):164A [A, B]

166. Woodman CL, Noyes R: Panic disorder: treatment with valproate. J Clin Psychiatry 1994; 55:134–136 [B]

167. Munjack DJ, Crocker B, Cabe D, Brown R, Usigli R, Zulueta A, McManus M, McDowell D, Palmer R, Leonard M: Alprazolam, propranolol, and placebo in the treatment of panic disorder and agoraphobia with panic attacks. J Clin Psychopharmacol 1989; 9:22–27 [A]

168. Ravaris CL, Friedman MJ, Hauri PJ, McHugo GJ: A controlled study of alprazolam and propranolol in panic-disordered and agoraphobic outpatients. J Clin Psychopharmacol 1991; 11:344–350 [A]

169. Shehi M, Patterson WM: Treatment of panic attacks with alprazolam and propranolol. Am J Psychiatry 1984; 141:900–901 [B]

170. Klein E, Uhde TW: Controlled study of verapamil for treatment of panic disorder. Am J Psychiatry 1988; 145:431–434 [A]

171. Benjamin J, Levine J, Fux M, Aviv A, Levy D, Belmaker RH: Double-blind, placebo-controlled, crossover trial of inositol treatment for panic disorder. Am J Psychiatry 1995; 152:1084–1086 [A]

172. Uhde TW, Stein MB, Vittone BJ, Siever LJ, Boulenger JP, Klein E, Mellman TA: Behavioral and physiologic effects of short-term and long-term administration of clonidine in panic disorder. Arch Gen Psychiatry 1989; 46:170–177 [A, B]

173. Spielberger CD: State-Trait Anxiety Inventory. Palo Alto, Calif, Consulting Psychologists Press, 1985 [G]

174. Zung WWK: A rating instrument for anxiety disorders. Psychosomatics 1971; 12:371–379 [G]

175. Hoehn-Saric R, Merchant AF, Keyser ML, Smith VK: Effects of clonidine on anxiety disorders. Arch Gen Psychiatry 1981; 38:1278–1282 [B]

176. Sheehan DV, Raj AB, Harnett-Sheehan K, Soto S, Knapp E: The relative efficacy of high-dose buspirone and alprazolam in the treatment of panic disorder: a double-blind placebo-controlled study. Acta Psychiatr Scand 1993; 88:1–11 [A]

177. Sheehan DV, Raj A, Sheehan KH, Soto S: Is buspirone effective for panic disorder? J Clin Psychopharmacol 1990; 10:3–11 [A]

178. Pollard CA: Inpatient treatment of complicated agoraphobia and panic disorder. Hosp Community Psychiatry 1987; 38:951–958 [B]

179. Pollard HJ, Pollard CA: Follow-up study of an inpatient program for complicated agoraphobia and panic disorder. Anxiety Disorders Practice J 1993; 1:37–40 [C]

180. Cottraux J, Note ID, Cungi C, Legeron P, Heim F, Chneiweiss L, Bernard G, Bouvard M: A controlled study of cognitive behaviour therapy with buspirone or placebo in panic disorder with agoraphobia. Br J Psychiatry 1995; 167:635–641 [A]

181. Wolfe BE, Maser JD (eds): Treatment of Panic Disorder: A Consensus Development Conference. Washington, DC, American Psychiatric Press, 1994 [G]

182. Coryell W, Noyes R, Clancy J: Excess mortality in panic disorder. Arch Gen Psychiatry 1982; 39:701–703 [D]

183. Noyes R: Suicide and panic disorder: a review. J Affect Disord 1991; 22:1–11 [F]

184. Warshaw MG, Massion AO, Peterson LG, Pratt LA, Keller MB: Suicidal behavior in inpatients with panic disorder: retrospective and prospective data. J Affect Disord 1995; 34:235–247 [C, D]

185. Lepine JP, Chignon M, Teherani M: Suicide attempts in patients with panic disorder. Arch Gen Psychiatry 1993; 50:144–149 [D]

186. Johnson J, Weissman MM, Klerman GL: Panic disorder comorbidity and suicide attempts. Arch Gen Psychiatry 1990; 47:805–808 [D]

187. Beck AT, Steer RA, Snaderson WC, Skeie TM: Panic disorder and suicidal ideation and behavior: discrepant findings in psychiatric outpatients. Am J Psychiatry 1991; 148:1195–1199 [D]

188. Hornig CD, McNally RJ: Panic disorder and suicide attempt: a reanalysis of data from the Epidemiologic Catchment Area study. Br J Psychiatry 1995; 167:76–79 [D]

189. Fawcett J, Scheftner WA, Fogg L, Clark DC, Young MA, Hedeker D, Gibbons R: Time-related predictors of suicide in major affective disorder. Am J Psychiatry 1990; 147:1189–1194 [C]

190. Mannuzza S: Panic disorder and suicide attempts. J Anxiety Disord 1992; 6:261–274 [D]

191. Cox BJ, Direnfeld DM, Swinson RP, Norton GR: Suicidal ideation and suicide attempts in panic disorder and social phobia. Am J Psychiatry 1994; 151:882–887 [D]

192. Friedman S, Jones JC, Chernen L, Barlow DH: Suicidal ideation and suicide attempts among patients with panic disorder: a survey of two outpatient clinics. Am J Psychiatry 1992; 149:680–685 [D]

193. Kushner MG, Sher KJ, Beitman BD: The relation between alcohol problems and the anxiety disorders. Am J Psychiatry 1990; 147:685–695 [F]

194. Anthony JC, Tien AY, Petronis KR: Epidemiological evidence on cocaine use and panic attacks. Am J Epidemiol 1989; 129:543–549 [C]

195. Mirin SM, Weiss RD, Griffin ML, Michael JL: Psychopathology in drug users and their families. Compr Psychiatry 1991; 32:36–51 [E]

196. Nunes E, Quitkin B, Berman C: Panic disorder and depression in female alcoholics. J Clin Psychiatry 1988; 49:441–443 [F]

197. Aronson TA, Craig TJ: Cocaine precipitation of panic disorder. Am J Psychiatry 1986; 143:643–645 [D]

198. Pallanti S, Mazzi D: MDMA (Ecstasy) precipitation of panic disorder. Biol Psychiatry 1992; 32:91–95 [G]

199. Moran C: Depersonalization and agoraphobia associated with marijuana use. Br J Med Psychol 1986; 59:187–196 [B]

200. Cowley DS: Alcohol abuse, substance abuse, and panic disorder. Am J Med 1992; 92(suppl 1A):41S–48S [F]

201. Brown SA, Irwin M, Schuckit MA: Changes in anxiety among abstinent male alcoholics. J Stud Alcohol 1991; 52:55–61 [B]

202. Thevos AK, Johnston AL, Latham PK, Randall CL, Adinoff B, Malcolm R: Symptoms of anxiety in inpatient alcoholics with and without DSM-III-R anxiety diagnoses. Alcohol Clin Exp Res 1991; 15:102–105 [B]

203. George DT, Nutt DJ, Dwyer BA, Linnoila M: Alcoholism and panic disorder: is the comorbidity more than coincidence? Acta Psychiatr Scand 1990; 81:97–107 [F]

204. Cox BJ, Norton GR, Swinson RP, Endler NS: Substance abuse and panic-related anxiety: a critical review. Behav Res Ther 1990; 28:385–393 [E]

205. Anthenelli RM, Schuckit MA: Affective and anxiety disorders and alcohol and drug dependence: diagnosis and treatment. J Addict Dis 1993; 12:73–87 [F]

206. Tucker P, Westermeyer J: Substance abuse in patients with comorbid anxiety disorder. Am J Addictions 1995; 4:226–233 [C]

207. Westermeyer J, Tucker P: Comorbid anxiety disorder and substance disorder. Am J Addictions 1995; 4:97–106 [C]

208. Ciraulo DA, Sands BF, Shader RI: Critical review of liability for benzodiazepine abuse among alcoholics. Am J Psychiatry 1988; 145:1501–1506 [F]

209. Shelton RC, Harvey DS, Stewart PM, Loosen PT: Alprazolam in panic disorder: a retrospective analysis. Prog Neuropsychopharmacol Biol Psychiatry 1993; 17:423–434 [E]

210. Lucas PB, Pickar D, Kelsoe J, Rapaport M, Pato C, Hommer D: Effects of the acute administration of caffeine in patients with schizophrenia. Biol Psychiatry 1990; 28:35–40 [B]

211. Leibenluft E, Fiero PL, Bartko JJ, Moul DE, Rosenthal NE: Depressive symptoms and the self-reported use of alcohol, caffeine, and carbohydrates in normal volunteers and four groups of psychiatric outpatients. Am J Psychiatry 1993; 150:294–301 [E]

212. Boulenger J-P, Uhde TW, Wolff EA, Post RM: Increased sensitivity to caffeine in patients with panic disorder. Arch Gen Psychiatry 1984; 41:1067–1071 [D]

213. Bowen R, South M, Hawkes J: Mood swings in patients with panic disorder. Can J Psychiatry 1994; 39:91–94 [G]

214. Savino M, Perugi G, Simonini E, Soriani A, Cassano GB, Akiskal HS: Affective comorbidity in panic disorder: is there a bipolar connection? J Affect Disord 1993; 28:155–163 [D, G]

215. Marks IM: Fears, Phobias, and Rituals. New York, Oxford University Press, 1987 [G]

216. Marks IM: Agoraphobia, panic disorder and related conditions in the DSM-IIIR and ICD-10. J Psychopharmacol 1987; 1:6–12 [G]

217. Herve C, Gaillard M, Roujas F, Huguenard P: Alcoholism in polytrauma. J Trauma 1986; 26:1123–1126 [E]

218. Boudewyns PA, Woods MG, Hyer L, Albrecht JW: Chronic combat-related PTSD and concurrent substance abuse: implications for treatment of this frequent "dual diagnosis." J Trauma Stress 1991; 4:549–560 [D]

219. Davidson J, Kudler H, Smith R: Treatment of posttraumatic stress disorder with amitriptyline and placebo. Arch Gen Psychiatry 1990; 47:259–266 [A]

220. Davidson JR, Kudler HS, Saunders WB, Smith RD: Symptom and comorbidity patterns in World War II and Vietnam veterans with posttraumatic stress disorder. Compr Psychiatry 1990; 31:162–170 [D]

221. Pitman RK, Altman B, Greenwald E: Psychiatric complications during flooding therapy for posttraumatic stress disorder. J Clin Psychiatry 1991; 52:17–20 [G]

222. Dansky BS, Roitzsch JC, Brady KT, Saladin ME: Posttraumatic stress disorder and substance abuse: use of research in a clinical setting. J Trauma Stress 1997; 10:141–148 [C]

223. Cottler LB, Compton WM III, Mager D, Spitznagel EL, Janca A: Posttraumatic stress disorder among substance users from the general population. Am J Psychiatry 1992; 149:664–670 [E]

224. Greist JH, Jefferson JW: Panic Disorder and Agoraphobia: A Guide, 2nd revised ed. Middleton, Wis, Dean Foundation for Health, Research, and Education, 1993 [G]

225. Mavissakalian M: The relationship between panic disorder/agoraphobia and personality disorders. Psychiatr Clin North Am 1990; 13:661–684 [F]

226. Brooks RB, Baltazar PL, McDowell DE, Munjack DJ, Bruns JR: Personality disorders co-occurring with panic disorder with agoraphobia. J Personality Disorders 1991; 5:328–336 [D]

227. Pollack MH, Otto MW, Rosenbaum JF, Sachs GS: Personality disorders in patients with panic disorder: association with childhood anxiety disorders, early trauma, comorbidity, and chronicity. Compr Psychiatry 1992; 33:78–83 [C]

228. Reich JH: DSM-III personality disorders and the outcome of treated panic disorder. Am J Psychiatry 1988; 145:1149–1152 [B]

229. Reich J, Troughton E: Frequency of DSM-III personality disorders in patients with panic disorder: comparison with psychiatric and normal control subjects. Psychiatry Res 1988; 26:89–100 [A]

230. Reich JH, Vasile RG: Effect of personality disorders on the treatment outcome of axis I conditions: an update. J Nerv Ment Dis 1993; 181:475–484 [F]

231. Green M, Curtis GC: Personality disorders and panic patients: response to termination of antipanic medication. J Personal Disord 1988; 2:303–314 [B]

232. Chambless DL, Renneberg B, Goldstein A, Gracely EJ: MCMI-diagnosed personality disorders among agoraphobic outpatients: prevalence and relationship of severity and treatment outcome. J Anxiety Disord 1992; 6:195–211 [D]

233. Marchand A, Goyer LR, Mainguy N: L'impact de la presence de troubles de la personnalité sur la réponse au traitement behavioral-cognitif du trouble panique avec agoraphobie. Science et Comportement 1992; 22:149–161 [B]

234. Black DW, Wesner RB, Gabel J, Bowers W, Monahan P: Predictors of short-term treatment response in 66 patients with panic disorder. J Affect Disord 1994; 30:233–241 [A]

235. Dreessen L, Arntz A, Luttels C, Sallaerts S: Personality disorders do not influence the results of cognitive behavioral therapies for anxiety disorders. Compr Psychiatry 1994; 35:265–274 [B]

236. Keijsers GPJ, Hoogduin CAL, Schapp CPDR: Prognostic factors in the behavioral treatment of panic disorder with and without agoraphobia. Behavior Therapy 1994; 25:689–708 [B]

237. Karajgi B, Rifkin A, Doddi S, Kolli R: The prevalence of anxiety disorders in patients with chronic obstructive pulmonary disease. Am J Psychiatry 1990; 147:200–201 [D]

238. Kaplan DS, Masand PS, Gupta S: The relationship of irritable bowel syndrome (IBS) and panic disorder. Ann Clin Psychiatry 1996; 8:81–88 [D]

239. Lydiard RB, Greenwald S, Weissman MM, Johnson J, Drossman DA, Ballenger JC: Panic disorder and gastrointestinal symptoms: findings from the NIMH Epidemiologic Catchment Area project. Am J Psychiatry 1994; 151:64–70 [E]

240. Kawachi I, Colditz GA, Ascherio A, Rimm E, Giovannucci E, Stampfer MJ, Willett WC: Prospective study of phobic anxiety and risk of coronary heart disease in men. Circulation 1994; 89:1992–1997 [C]

241. American Academy of Child and Adolescent Psychiatry: Practice Parameters for the Assessment and Treatment of Children and Adolescents With Anxiety Disorders. J Am Acad Child Adolesc Psychiatry 1997; 36(10 suppl):69S–84S [G]

242. Black B: Separation anxiety disorder and panic disorder, in Anxiety Disorders in Children and Adolescents. Edited by March J. New York, Guilford Press, 1995, pp 212–234 [G]

243. Black B, Robbins D: Panic disorder in children and adolescents. J Am Acad Child Adolesc Psychiatry 1990; 29:36–44 [F]

244. Kearney CA, Silverman WK: The panic disorder controversy continues. J Am Acad Child Adolesc Psychiatry 1991; 30:852–853 [G]

245. Kearney CA, Silverman WK: Let's not push the "panic" button: a critical analysis of panic and panic disorder in adolescents. Clin Psychol Rev 1992; 12:293–305 [E]

246. Whitaker A, Johnson J, Shaffer D, Rapoport JL, Kalikow K, Walsh BT, Davies M, Braiman S, Dolinsky A: Uncommon troubles in young people: prevalence estimates of selected psychiatric disorders in a nonreferred adolescent population. Arch Gen Psychiatry 1990; 47:487–496 [D]

247. Hayward C, Killen JD, Hammer LD, Lift IF, Wilson DM, Simmonds B, Taylor CB: Pubertal stage and panic attack history in sixth- and seventh-grade girls. Am J Psychiatry 1992; 149:1239–1243 [D]

248. Curry J, Murphy L: Comorbidity of anxiety disorders, in Anxiety Disorders in Children and Adolescents. Edited by March J. New York, Guilford Press, 1995, pp 301–317 [G]

249. Kovacs M, Feinberg TL, Crouse-Novak MA, Paulauskas SL, Finkelstein R: Depressive disorders in childhood, I: a longitudinal prospective study of characteristics and recovery. Arch Gen Psychiatry 1984; 41:229–237 [B]

250. Bernstein GA: Comorbidity and severity of anxiety and depressive disorders in a clinic sample. J Am Acad Child Adolesc Psychiatry 1991; 30:43–50 [C]

251. Last CG, Francis G, Hersen M, Kazdin AE, Strauss CC: Separation anxiety and school phobia: a comparison using DSM-III criteria. Am J Psychiatry 1987; 144:653–657 [D]

252. Last CG, Strauss CC: School refusal in anxiety-disordered children and adolescents. J Am Acad Child Adolesc Psychiatry 1990; 29:31–35 [D]

253. Gittelman-Klein R, Klein DF: School phobia: diagnostic considerations in the light of imipramine effects. J Nerv Ment Dis 1973; 156:199–215 [B]

254. Ollendick TH: Cognitive behavioral treatment of panic disorder and agoraphobia in adolescents: a multiple baseline design analysis. Behavior Therapy 1995; 26:517–531 [E]

255. Barlow DH: Effectiveness of behavior treatment for panic disorder with and without agoraphobia, in Treatment of Panic Disorder: A Consensus Development Conference. Edited by Wolfe BE, Maser JD. Washington, DC, American Psychiatric Press, 1994, pp 105–120 [G]

256. Ballenger JC, Carek DJ, Steele JJ, Cornish-McTighe D: Three cases of panic disorder with agoraphobia in children. Am J Psychiatry 1989; 146:922–924 [G]

257. Biederman J: Clonazepam in the treatment of prepubertal children with panic-like symptoms. J Clin Psychiatry 1987; 48(Oct suppl):38–42 [B]

258. Birmaher B, Waterman GS, Ryan N, Cully M: Fluoxetine for childhood anxiety disorders. J Am Acad Child Adolesc Psychiatry 1994; 33:993–999 [B]

259. Kutcher SP, MacKenzie S: Successful clonazepam treatment of adolescents with panic disorder. J Clin Psychopharmacol 1988; 8:299–301 [G]

260. Blazer D, George LK, Hughes D: The epidemiology of anxiety disorders: an age comparison, in Anxiety and the Elderly: Treatment and Research. Edited by Salzman C, Lebowitz BD. New York, Springer, 1991, pp 17–30 [G]

261. Eaton WW, Dryman A, Weissman MM: Panic and phobia, in Psychiatric Disorders in America. Edited by Robins LN, Regier DA. New York, Free Press, 1991, pp 155–179 [G]

262. Altshuler LL, Cohen L, Szuba MP, Burt VK, Gitlin M, Mintz J: Pharmacologic management of psychiatric illness during pregnancy: dilemmas and guidelines. Am J Psychiatry 1996; 153:592–606 [F]

263. Regier DA, Myers JK, Kramer M, Robins LN, Blazer DG, Hough RL, Eaton WW, Locke BZ: The NIMH Epidemiologic Catchment Area program: historical context, major objectives, and study population characteristics. Arch Gen Psychiatry 1984; 41:934–941 [G]

264. Kessler RC, McGonagle KA, Zhao S, Nelson CB, Hughes M, Eshleman S, Wittchen HU, Kendler KS: Lifetime and 12 month prevalence of DSM-III-R psychiatric disorders in the United States: results from the National Comorbidity Survey. Arch Gen Psychiatry 1994; 51:8–19 [C]

265. Blazer D, George LK, Landerman R, Pennybacker M, Melville ML, Woodbury M, Manton KG, Jordan K, Locke B: Psychiatric disorders: a rural/urban comparison. Arch Gen Psychiatry 1985; 42:651–656; correction 1986; 43:1142 [G]

266. Horwath E, Johnson J, Hornig CD: Epidemiology of panic disorder in African-Americans. Am J Psychiatry 1993; 150:465–469 [D]

267. Paradis CM, Friedman S, Lazar RM, Grubea J, Kesselman M: Use of a structured interview to diagnose anxiety disorders in a minority population. Hosp Community Psychiatry 1992; 43:61–64 [G]

268. Bell CC, Shakoor B, Thompson B, Dew D, Hughley E, Mays R, Shorter-Gooden K: Prevalence of isolated sleep paralysis in black subjects. J Natl Med Assoc 1984; 76:501–508 [D]

269. Neal AM, Smucker WD: The presence of panic disorder among African American hypertensives: a pilot study. J Black Psychol 1994; 20:29–35 [D]

270. Bell CC, Hildreth CJ, Jenkins EJ, Carter C: The relationship of isolated sleep paralysis and panic disorder to hypertension. J Natl Med Assoc 1988; 80:289–294 [D]

271. Brown C, Schulberg HC, Madonia MJ: Clinical presentations of major depression by African Americans and whites in primary medical care practice. J Affect Disord 1996; 41:181–191 [A]

272. Neighbors HW: Seeking help for personal problems: black Americans' use of health and mental health services. Community Ment Health J 1985; 21:156–166 [D]

273. Cooper-Patrick L, Crum RM, Ford DE: Characteristics of patients with major depression who received care in general medical and specialty mental health settings. Med Care 1994; 32:15–24 [E]

Category 1 Continuing Medical Education Credit for Practice Guideline for the Treatment of Patients With Panic Disorder

The American Psychiatric Association (APA) is pleased to offer you Continuing Medical Education (CME) credit for your participation in this practice guideline study program.

Practice guidelines are patient care strategies developed to assist physicians in clinical decision making. They are developed based on the degree of public importance, relevance to psychiatric practice, availability of information and relevant data, availability of work already done that could be useful in its development, and degree to which increased psychiatric attention in that area would be helpful to the field. Enduring materials developed under practice guidelines meet the needs of advancing clinical knowledge and enriching and expanding the skills of APA members with the ultimate goal of improving patient care.

Readers of *Practice Guideline for the Treatment of Patients With Panic Disorder* who wish to earn CME Category 1 credit may do so by answering the CME questions on the tear-out Answer Sheet at the back of the guideline.

The CME activity was planned and produced in accordance with the Essentials of the Accreditation Council for Continuing Medical Education.

The APA is accredited by the Accreditation Council for Continuing Medical Education (ACCME) to sponsor continuing medical education for physicians.

The APA designates this educational activity for 3.0 hours in Category 1 credit toward the Physician's Recognition Award of the American Medical Association and for the CME requirement of the APA. Each physician should claim only those hours of credit that he/she actually spent in the educational activity.

Target audience	Clinicians who treat patients with panic disorder; psychiatrists interested in the latest research findings and clinical applications in the treatment of panic disorder
Estimated time to complete	3 hours
Date of original release	May 1998
Next program evaluation date	May 2001
Program end date	May 2003

Principal faculty

There was no support from commercial sources used in the development and production of this CME product.

John S. McIntyre, M.D.—Chair, Department of Psychiatry, St. Mary's Hospital; Clinical Professor of Psychiatry, University of Rochester. Dr. McIntyre has no financial interest in or affiliation with any commercial supporter of these educational activities and/or providers of commercial services discussed in the guideline.

Deborah A. Zarin, M.D.—Deputy Medical Director, American Psychiatric Association. Dr. Zarin is employed by the American Psychiatric Association, who authored the practice guideline.

Jack Gorman, M.D.—Professor of Psychiatry, Columbia University; Deputy Director, New York Psychiatric Institute. Dr. Gorman has received grant support from SmithKline Beecham, Pfizer, Lilly, Bristol-Meyers Squibb, and Interneuron; serves on the speakers' bureau for Lilly, Bristol-Meyers Squibb, and SmithKline Beecham; and is on the advisory boards of Lilly, SmithKline Beecham, Pfizer, Forrest, Wyeth Ayerst, and Bristol-Meyers Squibb.

Katherine Shear, M.D.—Professor of Psychiatry, University of Pittsburgh; Director of Anxiety Disorders Prevention Program at Western Psychiatric Institute and Clinic/UPMC. Dr. Shear has received research grant support from Lilly, Pfizer, and SmithKline Beecham; serves on the speakers' bureau for Upjohn, SmithKline Beecham, Pfizer, and Hoffman LaRoche; and is a consultant with Pfizer, Glaxo, Hoffman LaRoche, SmithKline Beecham, and Bristol-Myers Squibb.

Educational objectives

- To acquaint physicians with the APA *Practice Guideline for the Treatment of Patients With Panic Disorder*
- To improve patient care for panic disorder by incorporating the principles of this guideline into individual practices

CME QUESTIONS
designated for 3 hours of CME Category 1 credit

1. Phenomenologically, panic attacks are discrete periods of intense fear or discomfort which usually peak in
   a. 2 minutes
   b. 10 minutes
   c. 40 minutes
   d. 60 minutes

2. The differential diagnosis for patients endorsing episodes of panic commonly includes the following except
   a. Posttraumatic stress disorder
   b. Separation anxiety disorder
   c. Alzheimer's disease
   d. Benzodiazepine withdrawal
   e. Hyperthyroidism

3. Which of the following can be present in a patient with panic disorder?
   a. Unexpected panic attacks
   b. Situationally bound attacks
   c. Nocturnal attacks
   d. Attacks associated with particular emotional contexts
   e. All of the above

4. The agoraphobia that may accompany panic disorder in some patients is typically marked by all of the following except
   a. Anxiety about places from which escape would be difficult
   b. Avoidance of places where the occurrence of a panic attack would prove difficult
   c. Curtailing of travel outside the home
   d. Impairment of occupational or personal interactions
   e. Fears of contamination

5. Which of the following is not true of panic disorder?
   a. Lifetime prevalence is approximately 2%
   b. Age at onset is in mid-life (40s to 50s)
   c. Risk is increased in females
   d. Depression is common in patients with panic

6. Which does not characterize patients with panic disorder?
   a. Increased risk of substance abuse
   b. Decreased risk of suicide attempts
   c. Increased risk of marital discord
   d. Increased use of psychoactive medication

The next four questions are TRUE OR FALSE:

7. Panic disorder shows a familial pattern.

8. Hospitalization frequently occurs to rule out a medical problem.

9. Approximately one-third of patients with panic disorder are depressed when they present for treatment.

10. Limited symptom attacks may occur before the clear onset of panic disorder and infrequently can occur prepubertally.

11. The frequent fear that panic attacks represent catastrophic medical events can be addressed with all of the following except
    a. Reassurance
    b. Education
    c. Enlisting familial support
    d. Encouraging phobic avoidance

12. The evaluation of a particular patient's panic symptoms can be aided by asking him or her to keep a journal; which details would be likely to be least helpful in characterizing the patient's panic experiences?
    a. Dates and times of the attacks
    b. Specific symptoms of each attack
    c. Emotional context surrounding each attack
    d. Length of treatment allowed by the patient's health plan
    e. Specific situations at the time of each attack

13. Evaluating the severity and nature of impairments can include
    a. Determining whether the attacks themselves or the anticipatory anxiety is more disruptive to the patient's life
    b. Eliciting what the patient defines as a satisfactory outcome
    c. Paying attention to familial or social arrangements that will be disrupted when the patient experiences symptomatic improvement
    d. All of the above

14. Which statement about the importance of maintaining a therapeutic alliance in the treatment of panic disorder is true?
    a. Panic disorder treatment is rarely long term.
    b. Patients are frequently asked to do frightening or difficult tasks.
    c. Patients are insensitive to separation from the psychiatrist.
    d. Patients are seldom anxious aside from their panic attacks.

15. The educational components of treatment of panic disorder can include
    a. Educating the patient that the symptoms do not represent a life-threatening medical illness
    b. Educating family members that panic disorder is a real illness that requires and responds to support and treatment

c. Educating nonpsychiatric physicians that panic attacks can easily masquerade as many other general medical conditions
d. Educating nonpsychiatric physicians that once the important, treatable general medical conditions have been ruled out, there is little to be gained from extensive medical testing
e. All of the above

16. When used for the treatment of panic disorder, cognitive-behavioral therapy (CBT) employs the following except

a. Education about the symptoms and the illness
b. Monitoring of symptoms
c. Anxiety management techniques, such as breathing exercises
d. Examination of the symbolic meaning of the symptoms
e. Exposure to fear cues

17. Components of "cognitive restructuring" as part of CBT include all the following except

a. Identifying and countering fears of bodily sensations
b. Identifying the likely bodily origin of feared sensations
c. Reshaping the estimation of the probability that a sensation represents a catastrophic medical illness
d. Interpreting the childhood antecedents of fearful situations

18. Exposure to fear cues can involve all of the following except

a. Developing a hierarchy of fear-evoking situations
b. Avoidance of fear-evoking situations
c. Initial exposure to the least intense situations
d. "Flooding" with exposure to extremely stressful situations
e. Agoraphobic exposure in the actual situation

19. When psychodynamic psychotherapy is used for treating panic disorder, which of these elements of psychic conflict come to be better understood and reintegrated in a more realistic and adaptive manner?

a. Impulses
b. Excessively harsh conscience and internal standards
c. Psychological defensive patterns
d. Realistic concerns
e. All of the above

20. The expected benefits of using selective serotonin reuptake inhibitors (SSRIs) in the treatment of panic disorder include

a. Reducing the intensity and frequency of panic attacks
b. Reducing anticipatory anxiety
c. Treating associated depression
d. All of the above

21. SSRI agents that have been investigated for use in panic disorder include all of the following except

   a. Fluoxetine (Prozac)
   b. Sertraline (Zoloft)
   c. Paroxetine (Paxil)
   d. Imipramine (Tofranil)
   e. Fluvoxamine (Luvox)

22. Side effects of SSRI medications that may be problematic in patients with panic disorder include all of the following except

   a. Irritability and increased anxiety
   b. Nausea and other gastrointestinal complaints
   c. Sexual dysfunction
   d. Tremor
   e. All of the above

23. The primary goals of benzodiazepine therapy for panic disorder include all of the following except

   a. To reduce the intensity and frequency of panic attacks
   b. To reduce anticipatory anxiety
   c. To reduce phobic avoidance
   d. To treat coexisting depression

24. Benzodiazepine medications that have been used to treat panic disorder include all of the following except

   a. Alprazolam (Xanax)
   b. Clonazepam (Klonopin)
   c. Topiramate (Topamax)
   d. Diazepam (Valium)
   e. Lorazepam (Ativan)

25. Factors that may complicate the use of benzodiazepine medications include

   a. Withdrawal symptoms or symptomatic rebound on discontinuation
   b. Memory complaints
   c. Fall risk in elderly patients
   d. Sedation
   e. All of the above

26. The group of medications with the least documented usefulness in the treatment of uncomplicated panic disorder is

   a. Anticonvulsant medications
   b. MAO inhibitors
   c. Serzone, nefazodone, and other atypical antidepressants
   d. Conventional neuroleptic medications
   e. Beta-adrenergic blocking agents

The next 10 questions are TRUE OR FALSE:

27. Patients with panic disorder and without depression routinely require inpatient hospitalization.

28. The treatment of panic disorder may be modified by the presence of a coexisting substance dependence disorder.

29. Because they do not understand the nature of panic disorder, family members may accuse the patient of overreacting and malingering.

30. If a patient becomes overly dependent on the psychiatrist, the dependency should be addressed directly and nonjudgmentally in the treatment, rather than through physician unavailability.

31. Available studies do not consistently demonstrate a superior efficacy of pharmacotherapy or of cognitive behavioral therapy for nonselected patient populations.

32. Because many patients with panic disorder are frequently highly sensitive to antidepressant medications at treatment initiation, it is recommended that doses approximately half of those given depressed patients to start treatment be employed for patients with panic disorder at the beginning, with titration as tolerated.

33. Tricyclic, SSRI, and monoamine oxidase inhibitor (MAOI) medications generally take 10–12 days to become effective for panic disorder.

34. Comorbid lifetime major depression, alcohol or substance abuse or dependence, personality disorders, brief depressive symptoms, and a history of suicide attempts increase the risk of suicide attempts in patients with panic disorder.

35. Approximately 40%–50% of patients with the diagnosis of panic disorder additionally meet criteria for one or more Axis II disorders.

36. Panic and other anxiety disorders are less prevalent in medically ill patients than in the population at large.

33) False, 34) True, 35) True, 36) False
27) False, 28) True, 29) True, 30) True, 31) True, 32) True,
18) b, 19) e, 20) d, 21) d, 22) e, 23) d, 24) c, 25) e, 26) d,
9) True, 10) True, 11) d, 12) d, 13) d, 14) b, 15) e, 16) d, 17) d,
Answers: 1) b, 2) c, 3) e, 4) e, 5) b, 6) b, 7) True, 8) True,

ANSWER SHEET

Please read the *Practice Guideline for the Treatment of Patients With Panic Disorder* carefully, then mark the correct answers to the 36 questions on this tear-out form. Complete the personal information required, and return it with your payment of $30 (CME processing fee) to Office of Education, American Psychiatric Association, 1400 K Street, N.W., Washington, D.C. 20005. Make your check payable to American Psychiatric Association. This self-test will not be accepted for scoring/CME certification after May 2003.

1	a	b	c	d	
2	a	b	c	d	e
3.	a	b	c	d	e
4.	a	b	c	d	e
5.	a	b	c	d	
6.	a	b	c	d	
7.	T	F			
8.	T	F			
9.	T	F			
10.	T	F			
11.	a	b	c	d	
12.	a	b	c	d	e
13.	a	b	c	d	
14.	a	b	c	d	
15.	a	b	c	d	e
16.	a	b	c	d	e
17.	a	b	c	d	
18.	a	b	c	d	e
19.	a	b	c	d	e
20.	a	b	c	d	
21.	a	b	c	d	e
22.	a	b	c	d	e
23.	a	b	c	d	
24.	a	b	c	d	e
25.	a	b	c	d	e
26.	a	b	c	d	e
27.	T	F			

28.	T	F
29.	T	F
30.	T	F
31.	T	F
32.	T	F
33.	T	F
34.	T	F
35.	T	F
36.	T	F

Evaluation of the Practice Guideline and CME Self-Study Activity

Please indicate your reaction to the following statements about this practice guideline and CME self-study activity by circling the appropriate response.

1. Overall, the quality of the practice guideline and study questions is excellent.
   - A. Strongly agree
   - B. Agree
   - C. Disagree
   - D. Strongly disagree

2. The practice guideline and study questions met their stated objectives.
   - A. Strongly agree
   - B. Agree
   - C. Disagree
   - D. Strongly disagree

3. The practice guideline and study questions provide information that I find useful for my practice.
   - A. Strongly agree
   - B. Agree
   - C. Disagree
   - D. Strongly disagree

4. The APA practice guidelines are useful for teaching.
   - A. Strongly agree
   - B. Agree
   - C. Disagree
   - D. Strongly disagree

5. The APA practice guidelines are useful for treating patients.
   - A. Strongly agree
   - B. Agree
   - C. Disagree
   - D. Strongly disagree

I certify that I have read this material and studied the questions for a total of at least 3 hours.

_____
Signature

_____
Name

_____
Address

_____
Daytime phone

_____
Fax

Are you an APA member?   ❐ **YES**   ❐ **NO**

_____
APA Member Number or Social Security Number

❐ **Check enclosed for $30 (CME processing fee)**
   (made payable to American Psychiatric Association)

Charge my   ❐ **Visa**   ❐ **MasterCard**

_____
Card number/Expiration date

_____
Signature

Return completed form with payment of $30 to

American Psychiatric Association
Office of Education
1400 K Street, N.W.
Washington, D.C. 20005

Program End Date: May 2003 (Self-test will not be accepted for scoring/CME certification after this date.)